AdM Home Care Coaching

FAMILY GUIDE TO IMPROVED HEALTH

DR. ROBERT E. WRIGHT
Ph.D., MHA, MA, RN
AND
CHRISTOPHER PREISLER

Behavior is what a man does. It is not what he thinks, feels, or believes.

— EMILY DICKINSON 1830-1886

Printed in the United States of America

First Printing: April 2020

Behavioral Education and Research Services, Inc.

ISBN (Print Edition): 978-1-09831-221-3

ISBN (eBook Edition): 978-1-09831-222-0

I want to thank my friend and colleague, Christopher Preisler, for attempting to dissect my many years of applied behavioral experience to put them down in such a readable form.

I would also like to express my most profound appreciation to our wives, who put up with many years of a very thin variable schedule of positive reinforcement from us!

Bob Wright

Adherence Management (AdM) Home Coaching: Family Guide To Improved Health

Over my MANY years in nursing and as an audiologist, I cared for countless people and their endless array of illnesses and injuries. For the young and middle-aged, normal health is pretty much on automatic pilot. There are many colds, an occasional touch of flu, scrapes, bruises, a broken bone or two, and a few sutures to ensure wounds heal properly. Others have challenges with early-onset chronic illnesses such as diabetes or epilepsy. Still others lay the foundation for future chronic diseases by engaging in behaviors of smoking, drug use, over-eating, excessive drinking, and a lack of physical exercise.

Many years ago, Dr. Ivar Lovaas was fond of saying, "All behavior returns to baseline." Baselines are the habits we form and the lifestyles we live. Taking pills, following restrictive diets, and exercising daily typically are not behaviors of our youth. They are not the baseline of habits necessary to achieve or maintain optimum health. As we approach middle age, the rituals required to follow a medical care plan are not in our book of life.

As you will read later in this book, most new behaviors needed to stave off bad habits or overcome genetic predispositions are not reinforcing. My colleague and friend Dr. Aubrey Daniels is fond of saying, "Behavior goes where reinforcement flows." On the surface, nothing is reinforcing about taking a handful of pills. Medications can be inconvenient, expensive, and confusing. On top of that, some side-effects may make us feel sick while our disease may not have any symptoms. It is understandable why people give up taking pills.

You Are Not Alone.

In my early 30s, I was visited by a kidney stone and was introduced to bloody urine and enough pain to get my attention. The stone passed, and I was fixed. Over the next several decades, there were several more stone episodes to remind me that I was not super-human. I was human. On a 2003 return trip from Washington, DC to Dallas, I noticed a small amount of particular pain in my left shoulder. There was not the crushing sensation that I had seen in so many patients during my ER years. There was no profuse sweating, but I called my family practice doctor as I waited for my wife to pick me up. His advice was direct. Go to the ER; do not go home. I went to the ER, and one of my nurse colleagues greeted me and escorted me to an exam room. Cardiac enzymes were drawn, an IV was started, and I was comfortably uncomfortable. My nurse colleague advised me that my troponin level was high, and I was admitted to the CCU. The next morning, I had my first stent put in. That was 18 years ago.

I continued my regular exercises, coached ice hockey, and remained in excellent health. The following year we relocated to Orlando, Florida. As the years passed, I heeded my cardiologist's advice and followed his medication regimen without missing a dose. Despite that, I had another two stents placed. On discharge each time, I filled my prescriptions and maintained my strict adherence to his plan of care.

I was the ideal patient. In fact, if you ask most physicians, they might tell you most of their patients are adherent. But with all due respect to their observations, studies show that more than 80% of all patients become non-adherent within a month or two after they are discharged from the hospital. Unless physicians are "cherry-picking" and "lemon dropping" their patients, at least half of them do not and will not follow their care plan. This book was written to recommend evidence-based methods for improving the behaviors of people who follow their care plans and for supporting family members who want the best for their "patient" once they come home from the hospital or care facility.

What Is A Patient?

"Patient" is a beautiful term that goes back to the early days of medicine several thousand years ago. The average patient is in the hospital less than a week, and then they are back to being whoever he or she was before they were tagged with the word "patient." Another of Dr. Aubrey Daniels' often used quotes is, "Past performance is the best indicator of future performance." What that means is you or your family member is no longer a "patient" once you return home. You are once again who you were before the health community labeled you. Your lifetime of habits are still there. You are returning to the very environment that may have contributed to your illness.

Our best clinicians have patched you up. You have met the criteria and time limit for this hospitalization. As the great writer Mark Twain (Samuel Clemmons) stated back in the 19th Century, the hospital "…tossed you out the window." His statement's full text is, "Habit is habit and not to be tossed out the window by any man but, coaxed downstairs one step at a time." Understanding Mr. Twain and relating it to the period after discharge from the hospital, is the essence of adherence management. If, as clinicians, we handed you a prescription and a care plan and sent you on your way, we have figuratively "tossed you out the window."

Developing new habits requires, as the first step in this coaxing process, patient and family education. Further steps must be continued each day as new behaviors develop into adherent habits as outlined in the adherence improvement plan. There must also be sources of behavior reinforcement for the discharged "patient" and their supporting family members. A few minutes of "patient education" within moments of discharge and a handful of prescriptions and instructions to follow when you get home, does not a habit make!

The Patient's Perspective.

In September 2017, I was in Dallas for a week. I continued my daily walking in the hill country with no episodes of discomfort or shortness of breath. Then, in January 2018, I began to notice a slight bit of pain in my shoulder when I walked up the small incline approaching our home in Florida. My shoulder was not a problem, I thought. I knew I had an appointment with my cardiologist in a couple of days. On my appointment day, I mentioned the discomfort. He cut our time short and directed that I return in the morning for a heart cath. I checked in at the appointed time, and, as is usual, I declined a sedative. I preferred to watch the procedure on the screen. My doctor, always the consummate professional, completed the procedure without incident and advised me that he found an area of concern in one of my arteries. Since I had had several stents, and this was a Thursday, I asked if he was going to place another stent on Friday. "No, it's not in an area I'm comfortable stenting. I'm admitting you to the hospital." The weekend was fast approaching, and I asked if I should plan on a Monday admission. "No, you are going to be directly admitted as soon as we can get you to the hospital. I'm scheduling you for a two-vessel cabbage." (Coronary artery bypass graft - CABG) . It was Thursday, March 1, 2018.

No one can be sure of what might have happened during the almost 20 years between my first stent and this visit. I was confident in the reality that my adherence to the medication regimen likely contributed to the fact that I had not had a lethal event during that time. As a long-time nurse and clinician, I had concerns, but I was not overly worried. Within a short time, I would be in the cardiac care unit and monitored. I suppose I should have been afraid. I was not. I had a respectable level of concern. In my early career in nursing, I had been a cardiac ICU nurse. I assisted the recovery of numerous fresh CABGs, and now, forty years later, I was confident the bugs had been worked out over tens of thousands of procedures. My surgeon had an excellent reputation. As I spoke with the nurses in CCU and mentioned who my surgeon was, they all agreed they would want him to do their procedure.

I'll spare you the details of the day-to-day events that lasted from Thursday until my surgery early on a Sunday morning. I met my surgeon early Saturday evening as he was headed home from finishing several CABGs that day. Our conversation was both professional and cordial. Most importantly, I knew he was going home early, and I would be his first case on Sunday. Sunday morning came, and there were the expected pre-surgery activities as I was transported to pre-op. My best friend and wife walked with me as I was wheeled into pre-op and stayed with me as the IV was inserted, blood pressure and other vital signs monitored. The anesthesiologist introduced himself, and the word came from the OR that the team was ready. Everyone was in place, except for me. My pre-op nurse was fabulous as she was professional, friendly, and supportive. I kissed Jude Ann as she gave me a brave smile, and the last thing I remember was going through the pre-op doors en route to the operating room.

I woke up sometime later, thinking that wasn't too bad. I had no pain and was resting comfortably in the room where I would spend the next several days. Jude Ann and my youngest son Jefferson were in the room as I commented on how quickly the procedure went. Jefferson was the first to point out that it was now early Tuesday afternoon. I smiled and wondered what had happened to Sunday and Monday? The only proof anything out of the ordinary occurred was a photograph of me in the recovery ICU. I also had a new scar in the middle of my chest.

Patient Education.

My nursing care and clinician follow-up were superb. Nurses and nursing students, x-ray, and lab technicians washed their hands on entering and exiting my room. There was no doubt they were giving me the right medications as they checked my ID on every medication pass. Social workers, nurse clinicians, discharge planners, and nurse educators came in as scheduled to ensure that I had the things and information I needed to be successful. The days after my surgery were pretty routine. On Tuesday, mid-day, I received word that I might be discharged as early as Wednesday. Now that was an eye-opener for an old ICU nurse recovering CABG patients back in the mid-1970s. I was on my second postoperative day, and we were discussing discharge on the third day. My head was spinning as I looked back at my CABG nursing days. Patients came to the ICU in the late afternoon. We did all the necessary monitoring and used titrated morphine to keep them very quiet and intubated for at least 24 hours. If patients were stable on the second postoperative day, they were extubated and allowed to sit up and dangle their legs over the edge of the bed. By the third post-op day, we considered transferring them to the cardiac progressive care unit, and seven days later, they were candidates for discharge. I laughed to myself in comparing a 3rd post-op day discharge as my wife and I walked the hospital's halls. Times had changed.

As it turned out, I was discharged on the 6th postoperative day. There was a flurry of activity as patient education staff came in. They had an inch of materials to share with me. They talked about what had occurred and what I needed to do at home. There was a ton of information, reduced to a few ounces because of my years of experience. For the regular, non-medical patient, this volume of information must be like learning Swahili in a few easy lessons. There were follow-up appointments to make and keep with my surgeon, chest x-rays, prescriptions, cardiac rehab, and calls from follow-up nurses. There was also wound care for the chest incision, two chest tube incisions, and the two incisions from the vein donor site.

While none of this was overwhelming to me, I tried to envision this tsunami of information from the patients' perspective and the people tasked with supporting their sick family members. "Now this is important…" and then "This is important." It seemed that everything was essential or something terrible would happen. When everything is necessary, which behavior or symptom was the most important? It appeared that each specialty area thought his or her information was more important than the other. One of the primary causes of non-adherence is "confusion." Once again, as a long-time nurse, I was able to filter the mixed signals. I wondered what filters non-medical people might develop and if those filters might become harmful. Trust is essential in health services. Another primary cause of non-adherence is "distrust." Mixed signals or conflicting signals, real or perceived by patients is sufficient to lead to non-adherence. How would family members and patients resolve their issues of distrust or confusion when they arose?

Follow-up Care.

One of the more concerning issues with post-discharge care that goes beyond the actual clinical care is ensuring patients are not readmitted to the hospital within thirty days of discharge. The bureaucratic concern from US Congress authors of the Affordable Care Act of 2010 was ensuring there was a reduction in harm to patients in hospitals. Another goal was to ensure patients did not return to the hospital for unplanned readmission after they were discharged. Hospital nurses called me three times after I went home to check on my status. While I was pleased to have a conversation with them, they had no way of knowing whether or not I was an "at-risk" patient for becoming non-adherent. No tools or surveys were used on my admission to identify my risk factors. There was also no review of my discharge plan to see if there were any potential obstacles or "punishers" in the plan. These consequences could contribute to my abandoning the care plan. Without having a chance to identify these punishers, there would be no chance of having a conversation with my doctor about alternate plans that may have been more successful.

My nurses asked if I was going along with my care plan. "Of course," I said yes, and I was following my care plan. I was also reminded of one early admonition of Hippocrates to his students in the 4th Century BCE, "Keep a watch also on the faults of patients, which also make them lie about the taking of things prescribed." Why you might ask, would patients or their families lie about taking their medications or following other parts of their care plan? For that matter, why would patients lie to their family members or make excuses about doing the very behaviors that could improve their health and perhaps extend their quality and quantity of life? The answers are found in the consequences of each act. Care plan consequences that are immediately punishing to patients, from their perspective, will be abandoned.

Clinical consequences that are good for patients and occur sometime in the future may be quickly abandoned if there is no intermittent reinforcement to create and maintain adherent habits. The Adherence Improvement Plan (AIP), when implemented, is based on the outcomes of the BEARS' Adherence Consequence Analysis (BACA). The AIP is the road map to adherence and improved health results.

The Cheshire Cat in *Alice in Wonderland* suggested that "If you don't know where you want to go, then it doesn't matter which path you take." Following a personalized plan of care is one path. Not following the plan is another. The Cat asked Alice, "Where do you want to go?" When she answered, "I don't know." "Then," said the Cat, "It really doesn't matter, does it?" When patients don't know what they want or need to do with their care plan, then it is up to their families to provide guidance, support, and positive reinforcement to keep them on the right path. Unlike in the world of Wonderland, it "really does matter" which path to take.

What This Means To You.

Over the past 18-months, I have watched transitional care nurses assist families as their loved one is readied for returning home from a skilled nursing facility. They have their O2 concentrators, wheelchairs, crutches, medications, appointment slips, and an endless array of things. The nurse carefully checks off each item to ensure it is either in the hands of the family or is waiting for them at home. A copy of the discharge checklist is provided to the family. Each pill being sent home is accounted for and signed off by both the nurse and family member. Appointment slips and prescriptions are placed in a folder, and the family unit is walked or wheeled to the front door, assisted into the waiting cars, and they are on their way. The faces of many novice "patient care providers," and their weak smiles do not cover the reality that awaits the patient when they get home. That they are moving towards an adventure in their wonderland for which they are ill-prepared. Wonderland will be filled with an environment of smells and sounds, the access of which will awaken their old habits. "I know it's bad for me, and I'll just have one with my coffee or beer."

Family members and patients are not experts at in-home care. Most people are neither "intellectually fluent" nor "practically fluent" in Adherence Management Home Care, and that's okay. We are all fluent at being us and maintaining the relationships we have. We have pre-hospital "tools" we have used successfully for years. We are spouses, parents, workers, car drivers, grocery and major expense item purchasers, and many other roles. With post-hospital care and chronic illness, the road to recovery requires a few new tools. This book provides these tools. The home healthcare team needs a coach. Like it or not, and prepared or not, you are that coach. AdM Home Coach is your guide for improving or at least maintaining where your "patient" was at discharge.

I am now approaching two years since my CABG and discharge. The hospital and my surgical team did their jobs. My post-discharge team did their job with the tools they had. In the four most populated states, New York, California, Florida, and Texas, in 2019, there were more than seven million hospital discharges. Every day of the week, 19,000 families are taking a loved one home in these four states alone. There are not enough transitional care and home health nurses to provide a lifetime of adherent behavior support. Crossing that threshold from patient to person means that with each passing day, there is significantly less contact with the formal health delivery system and more family involvement.

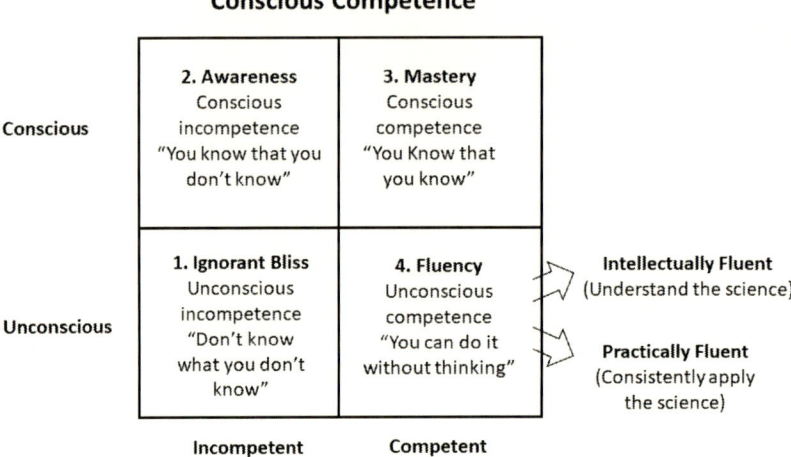

Four Categories Of Learning.

Chances are there is likely more positive reinforcement for not following the plan of care and more "punishers" for following the care plan. Will you know how to recognize and manage those threats to your loved one? There are four categories of learning when it comes to providing family home care. Before there is a chronic illness in the family, we are in group 1. We are in "Ignorant Bliss." All of us are in this state of "Unconscious Incompetence." There is nothing wrong with this condition. I am perfectly happy not knowing a lot of things until something happens.

When it comes to post-hospital care, a family member, or yourself, developed an illness, which you sought medical help to correct. You are about to be discharged, but you find yourself now in "Conscious Incompetence." This is where I frequently see families as their discharge approaches. They are aware of what needs to get done post-discharge, but I see the panic in the eyes and faces of too many of these people. There is a tremor in their voice and the fear that they will cause harm to their loved ones if they don't get everything just right. But it is more than just the clinical or care-taking components that bother them. "My husband hates taking medications. How can I get him to change?" AdM Home Coach will help you bridge the gap into the third box of "Conscious Competence." You can gain the skills needed to identify, shape, and reinforce adherent behavior. As time passes, you will achieve the fourth level, "Fluency." You will have "Unconscious – Competence." You will not have to think through every step to achieve the results you need. It is in this final stage where habits are formed and persistent patient adherence is born.

Good luck, and I look forward to hearing your story.

Table Of Contents

Introduction   1

   Specific Responsibilities And Tasks For Behavior Training.   2

American Health Services: Treating The Great ~~Melting~~ *Stew* Pot   5

   The Role Culture Plays In Healthcare.   6

   Other Approaches For Improving Adherence.   7

What Is Adherence Management   9

   AdM Coaching.   9

   #1 Secret To All Human Behavior   11

Behavioral Science   14

   What Is Behavior?   14

   My Patient Had No Behaviors Today.   15

   How To Describe Behavior-The Do's And Don'ts?   17

   Outcomes vs. Behaviors   18

   Behavior Must Be Described Without Using Labels.   19

   Desired Behavior (Label)   19

   Non-Adherent Behavior   21

   Why Do I Have To Know The Difference?   21

   Why Not Use "Good" And "Bad" In Describing Behavior?   22

   ABC's Of Behavior   22

   Why Do We Behave?   27

   Antecedents To Behavior.   29

   Why Focus So Much On What Happens Before The Behavior?   33

Consequences Of Behavior   35

   Consequences: What Happens After The Behavior?   36

   Consequences That Decrease Behavior.   37

   Punishment And Penalty   37

   An In-Depth Look At Consequences.   39

   Consequences That Increase Behavior.   39

   Increasing And Decreasing Behavior   40

What Is The Difference Between R- And P-?   41

Extinction   43

BEARS Adherence Consequence Analysis (BACA).   46

A Brief Look At How To Use BACA.   47

Consequences Are Described Using A Variety Of Terms.   49

Four Consequence Characteristic Category Pairs   52

The Complete Consequence Picture.   53

Strength Of A Consequence.   53

To Do or Not To Do.   54

Patient Centered Means Looking At Consequences From The Patient's Perspective.   55

Determine The Behaviors You Need For Success.   56

What May Happen If…   56

Antecedents In The BACA.   57

List All The Consequences   61

Determine Positive or Negative?   63

Determining Immediate or Future?   65

Determine Whether the Consequence is Likely or Unlikely To Occur?   68

Perception: Aware or Not Aware?   70

Seeing The Whole Picture.   73

What Does It All Mean?   73

Persistence vs. Extinction: The Long Haul Of Adherence   76

Can't Or Won't Behaviors   79

Human Repertoire.   81

The Ethics Of Behavior Change.   81

Reinforcement   83

Reinforcing Adherence – Getting Patients From Prescription To Persistence.   84

Reinforce The Behavior - Outcomes Will Follow   85

How Do We Determine What's Reinforcing?   86

Joy, Pleasure, Satisfaction – The Path To Meaningful Reinforcers.   87

Social And Tangible Reinforcers – Choosing The Right One.   88

Sacrifice And Satiation – Increasing And Decreasing The Value Of Reinforcers.   89

When Do I Give A Patient A Reinforcer?   91

Effectiveness Of Reinforcement.   93

Differential Reinforcement.   96

Documenting And Graphing Care Plans And Adherence Plans 98

Prompting Strategies 99

Graphing 101

Improvement Toward Adherence 103

Planning Better Outcomes With The "Some Of The Time" Patients. 103

Adherence Improvement Plan (AIP) 105

Can And Can't Reasons For Non-Adherence 105

Houston… We Have A Solution 106

I Won't Follow Your Recommendations Doctor… 107

Moving Won't To Will… When You Can 108

Pinpointing The Target Behavior 109

Whose Job Is It Anyway? 111

Adherence Improvement Plan (AIP) Page Two 113

Reinforcing The Target Behaviors 113

Positive Reinforcement. 113

Getting The Behavior Started And Maintaining It 116

Getting Patients On Board 116

AdM Home Coach Professionalism 119

Your Emotions 121

How Patients Interact With You. 122

What Do I Do If My Patient Is Not Cooperative? 123

What Do I Do When My Family Member Or Patient Engages In Adherent Behavior? 125

What Do I Do If What A Family Member Is Engaging In Non-Adherent Behavior? 126

Stop-Redirect-Reinforce Technique. 127

Evaluating When You Get Stuck 128

Common Reasons Adherence Fails 130

How Adherence Management Might Let You Down. 132

Limiting Your Care Plan Commitment. 132

Not Believing The Behavioral Process Is Evidence-Based. 133

No Investment In Coaching To Yield Habit-Strength. 134

I Thought An Introduction To Behavior Would Solve My Patient's Problems. 134

No Accountability Was Established. 135

Lifestyles Didn't Change… Did Not Incorporate R+. 136

No Investment In Training Home Based Coaches. 138

Thought That Education Alone Would Improve Adherence.   139

Thought They Knew More Than What 80+ Years Of Research Has Confirmed.   139

Epilogue: The AdM Home Coach Beginning   142

Appendix   144

Index   169

What's Your NEXT STEP? Telehealth!   172

Table of Appendix

Appendix A1: BEARS Adherence Consequence Analysis (BACA)   145

Appendix A2: BACA SAMPLE   146

Appendix B1: Adherence Improvement Plan (AIP) Page 1 Of 2   147

Appendix B2: Adherence Improvement Plan (AIP) Page 2 Of 2   148

Appendix C1: Baca For Beatriz.   149

Appendix C2: AIP For Beatriz   150

Appendix D: Dr. Wright's Evaluation Of "Losing Control."   151

Appendix E: Reinforcer Survey   156

Appendix F: Wright-Lindsley Review Process   157

Appendix G1: BEARS' Medical Adherence Assessment Scale (B-MAAS)   158

Appendix G2: B-MAAS, Instructions   159

Appendix H: BEARS' Physical Ability Assessment Scale (B-PAAS)   166

Appendix I: ABC Narrative And Training Worksheet   167

Introduction

Providing Adherence Management Coaching© (AdM Home Coach©) for patients and family members requires a knowledge of The Science of Behavior. My name is Dr. Bob Wright. I've been working directly with patients (and children & adults on the autism spectrum) for over 50 years. I have trained hundreds of direct support personnel, nurses, clinicians, CNAs, and facility administrators, but I wanted to write a book for anyone who takes care of people in their home environments. More and more health programs require post-care to be done in the home, but you may not know how to get your loved ones to do what the doctor ordered.

This training guide was developed to introduce you, both to the science of Applied Behavior Analysis and to the many tasks necessary to provide day-to-day activities in support of family members who need to make some behavior changes to create new habits after coming home from the hospital or rehab center. It is not a replacement for listening to your doctor or following their clinical directions. Caregivers reading this book will achieve better health results.

This book is the first step in the AdM Coach training series, which focuses on providing a baseline of information and then expanding clinical skills in Adherence Management Coaching©.

Specific Responsibilities And Tasks For Behavior Training.

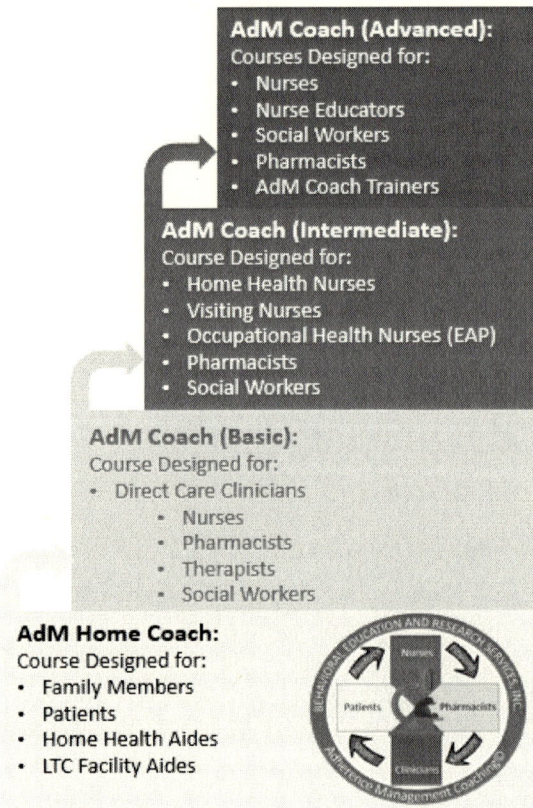

The Science of Behavior should be simple enough and presented at different levels so that every caregiver, person, or family member who works with patients have at least a basic understanding of how they can play their role. Consistency between providers and family members is essential for learning and producing the best possible outcomes for each patient. In this book, you will learn the role of the home caregiver.

The caregiver becomes the foundation for the overall Adherence Management Coaching program.

Up from the role of primary caregiver, you may want to move into a more professional role. To be effective as a Certified AdM Home Coach©, you will also need to complete at least the Introduction to Behavior training course to understand what is going on within the family member's adherence management program and understand why tasks are completed as they are. Our goal in the Introduction to Behavior course is to ensure Certified AdM Home Coaches©, are familiar with the concepts and language of Applied Behavior Analysis. In this course, you will learn the "Insider Secrets They Don't Teach You About Patient Adherence." The course consists of eight (8) hours of online instruction followed by a certification test. You will have instant credibility as one who "Pinpoints Consequences That Hinder, Reinforce Behaviors That Matter, and Celebrate Results That Change People's Lives."

For professional AdM Home Coaches© who work in homes with family members, this course is the minimum amount of training necessary to function safely and understand what is being done through the primary care clinician. It is essential that what is taught in the clinician's practice is continued into the home environment, whether the tasks are completed by clinic-based trainers or AdM Home Coaches©.

Once you move beyond the AdM Home Coach program, a more formal Masters Series training program is offered for clinicians, nurses, hospitals, long term care facilities, and other professional care providers. Each course builds on the knowledge gained from the previous level.

AdM Coach (Basics) is a 2-day training program that builds upon the AdM Home Coach program. It consists of more education related to The Science of Behavior and how to implement the Adherence Improvement Plan, and Educational Improvement plans developed for the certified AdM Home Coach.

AdM Coach (Intermediate level) is a 4.5-day training program that expands into working with physicians and behavioral scientists to implement the Adherence Improvement Plan (AIP) and document changes in behavior. The Intermediate AdM Coach© is a certified position, and providers must demonstrate a higher level of understanding of The Science of Behavior and how it relates to their profession, as well as how to integrate their specialty in a manner that ensures continuity between environments and providers.

AdM Coach (Advanced) training ensures that clinicians provide expert consultation and support to the entire treatment team. They are the team experts on the application of Adherence Management and coordinate all activities for each of the lower tiers. AdM Coach (Advanced) is an additional 4-day training program beyond the Intermediate AdM Coach level.

In this book, we will cover many of the skills and information necessary to understand The Science of Behavior and specific techniques that you can practice day-to-day to help your family members develop healthy habits. At the end of some sections, you will be given a list of key points that you should have learned in that section. As you master these skills, you should be prepared to be tested by AdM Coaches at higher levels than your own and demonstrate your expertise throughout your home coaching experience.

For clinicians to achieve certification at the AdM Coach (Advanced Level) entrance into the program requires successful completion of the Home, Basic and Intermediate echelons. To enter the Intermediate Level requires completion of AdM Home Coach and AdM Coach Basics levels. Certification as an AdM Home Coach involves completion of the Introduction to Adherence Management (8) Hour Module.

Adherence Management Coaching, at any level, is open to all interested health services professionals.

American Health Services:
Treating The Great ~~Melting~~ *Stew* Pot

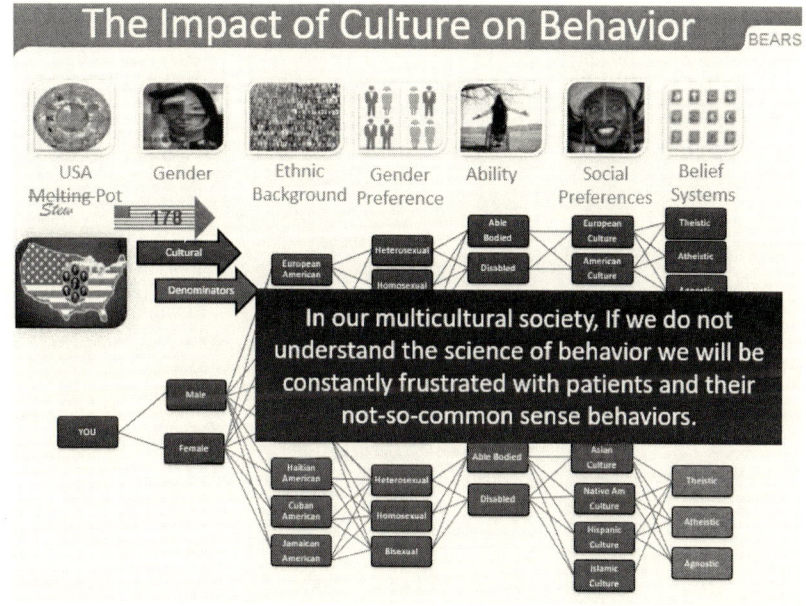

The common senses we all share were best defined by Aristotle (383 BCE): sight, hearing, taste, touch, and smell. Everything else we do is based on learned responses to specific antecedents (cues) in any given environment and the consequences we receive for those learned responses (behaviors.)

Hoping that "common sense" will prevail and people will do the "right thing" when it comes to their health and disease management has been the holy grail of health care since the beginning of recorded history. The very idea that all patients will follow medical advice and care plans because it makes common sense explains why non-adherence is so high. Families can only manage the care of their "patients" within the scope of their social norms.

During our lifetime, many habits will become part of our daily life. When disease interrupts that relative tranquility, health care providers disrupt our peace and quiet to have a brief encounter with us in their environments (the hospital or doctor's office), and then we return home to the climate that likely contributed to our disease state. We spend thousands of hours with friends, family and the internet, who all have opinions about how to treat every ailment. We see countless hours of drug commercials with their various warnings telling us all the possible side effects of the very prescription that our doctor just prescribed. All this bombardment of information counteracting the very messages we received during the short time we spent with our health services professional.

The Role Culture Plays In Healthcare.

Societies have always been a complex compilation of cultures and never more so than today. Large numbers of people from various cultures are being transplanted to the US, and for many, these transfers might occur in mere days or weeks. While biology is the same for all people, each culture brings its share of more than 170 habits, beliefs, and ways of doing things. They are rolled into the cultural stewpot known as the United States of America.

I say stewpot rather than melting pot because many people choose to maintain their cultures within pockets of American society rather than assimilate into traditional American culture. Each culture is bringing with it its own practices, languages, ways of dealing with illness, and countless habits. They may be uncommon to providers but very common to them. This concept is true for other countries as well. Whenever a group of people are displaced from one environment into one that is foreign to them, the group will try to maintain as much of the old culture as possible.

Social constructs and societies can be very complicated. Because of this, we think that human behavior must be equally complex. It is not. Understanding why people choose to follow their doctor's care plan or not is simple. This is why I wrote this book!

Other Approaches For Improving Adherence.

Over the past 100 years, three forms of traditional approaches to dealing with patient adherence have emerged: teachback, motivational interviewing, and medication therapy management.

First, **Teachback** focuses on providing patients with the appropriate information necessary to treat their disease and follow a plan of care. Patients and their families are introduced to new information related to their disease process and prescribed treatments. At various intervals, family members are requested to "teach-back" that information to the nurse educator to ensure they have a sufficient understanding of the new material.

Second, **Motivational Interviewing** is the approach to improving patient adherence by focusing on any ambivalence or feelings toward a disease and its treatment. Patients are described as having "wrong-thinking," and improved outcomes are the result of overcoming their previous knowledge by creating adherent thinking related to their disease process and prescribed treatments.

Third, **Medication Therapy Management** focuses on preventing harm by thoroughly reviewing all current and previous medications and any ingested substances (such as supplements or foods) for any possible drug interactions that can cause harm. Interactions are now usually completed automatically by clinicians or pharmacy technologies. However, this automated technology is only as good as the information fed into it. All prescriptions from every source must be entered. A patient may be receiving holistic medicines from their culture or eating foods that they believe are perfectly safe so they don't even mention it, but those same substances may adversely affect current treatments.

Our BRAND NEW APPROACH is Adherence Management (AdM) Coaching, which focuses on developing adherence habits. By understanding The Science of Behavior, family members and caregivers will identify those not-so-common sense behaviors and find ways to help the people they care for develop healthier habits to last a lifetime. Humans do the things they do because of what happens to them when they do it. Look at the consequences of what they do from their perspective. The primary function of this book is to help you understand why people do the things they do and how we can get more or less of those pinpointed behaviors that lead to healthier habits. Behavior is not what people think, feel or believe. Behavior is what people do!

What Is Adherence Management

Adherence Management Coaching© gets its foundations from the science of Applied Behavior Analysis. This evidence-based approach to behavior has been identified as the most effective treatment for individuals with autism and developmental disabilities. For more than 35 years, it has also been a useful tool in the workplace and is known as "Performance Management," by Dr. Aubrey Daniels.

The principles of Adherence Management Coaching are built upon these two great bodies of knowledge to apply it to the patient experience. It is used to teach tasks and skills to family members, caregivers, health care providers, and even healthcare administrators how to systematically reward adherent behaviors, stop rewarding non-adherent behavior, and providing support and positive reinforcement to transform adherence behaviors into new habits for maintaining health.

AdM Coaching.

AdM Coaching is an evidence-based, applied behavioral approach that methodically identifies patients who are "at-risk" for non-adherence by using the BEARS Medical Adherence Assessment Survey (see our B-MAAS assessment in Appendix G1).

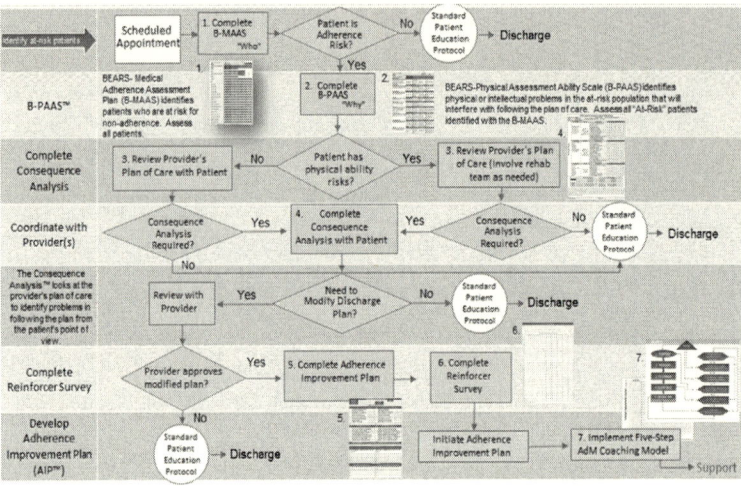

It then identifies if there are any physical or intellectual impairments that might contribute to an inability to follow a particular care plan by using the BEARS Physical Abilities Assessment Survey (see our B-PAAS assessment in Appendix H1).

A third component to AdM Coaching is looking at the discharge or care plan itself, from the patient's perspective, to identify related positive and negative consequences that could contribute to non-adherence. These consequences are then shared with the patient's physician. Where modifications can be made, providers can adjust the care plan. Where adjustments are not possible, a schedule of positive reinforcements are created to overcome any negative consequences in the plan of care.

The AdM Coach (nurse, pharmacist, transition care team) develops in Step 5 an Adherence Improvement Plan (AIP), and reviews it with the patient or their trained AdM Home Coach. Step 6 requires time to identify things and events that can be used as reinforcers as the AdM Coach helps shape new adherence habits. Step 7 uses the Wright-Lindsley Matrix (see Appendix F) to identify if progress towards adherence is being accomplished or whether modifications to the AIP are needed.

#1 Secret To All Human Behavior

The underlying assumption of the AdM Coach program is that we all behave or act as we do because of what happens to us when we do that behavior. For example, we order pizza because we expect the result will be a delivery person bringing a pizza to fill our need when we're hungry. We put money in the soda machine because we expect to hear the dropping of the bottle when we want a soda. We phone another person because we expect to get a person or answering machine at the other end when we want to talk to them. AdM Coaches learn that behavior is controlled or influenced by one thing: the consequences that are received after that behavior occurs. For example, what happens to your family member, as a direct result of their behavior, will either increase or decrease the likelihood that that behavior will occur again in the future. Whether or not it is an adherent behavior of following the care plan or non-adherent behavior that leads to unhealthy habits. It is the consequence of the behavior that drives the choice. Positive reinforcement increases behavior. Penalty and punishment decreases behavior.

In addition to teaching new skills or strengthening weak skills, AdM Home Coaches learn how to understand behavior and to figure out why their family members do the things they do. AdM Home Coaches also learn how their family member derive benefits from their non-adherent behaviors. And, why they perceive they are being punished for doing adherent behaviors, such as following their doctor's care plan.

They do this by recording information or data about behaviors, including things that happen in the environment before the adherent behavior and what things happen in the environment after the behavior. By figuring out the function of the family member's behavior, we can guide you as you make meaningful changes in your family member's life.

You may ask, "Why is this even important?" Long before becoming a patient, the family member spent years becoming the person they are. Upon discharge from a hospital or care clinic for the acute phase of their current illness, your patient will return to the same home environment and old habits that likely contributed to the very illness that caused the hospitalization. All these habits are waiting for them at home and work.

In the short time they were in the hospital or with clinical professionals in the various clinics; we expected them to learn how to deal with their illness and learn a repertoire of new skills and medical language. Then we want them to flawlessly execute their discharge plan or plan of care for weeks, months or even years to come. People with an acute illness may not be focusing on learning. They may not retain the information at all because all they are thinking about is getting out of the hospital.

For the most part, clinicians consider care plans as including simple tasks. However, family members or patients may not learn in the same manner. Post-discharge tasks can be very hard for the novice caregiver. Clinicians must learn to break down specific programs into minimal steps and teach (and reinforce) each step. Clinical tasks are often viewed as simple by clinicians. Yet they may be so complicated to the patient or caregiver so providers must encourage, help, and reinforce patients and their family members as they try to learn these steps and many other new skills. This is what an AdM Coach is all about. Spending time with patients to teach and reinforce new behaviors. Furthermore, while clinicians may be able to understand the information that they work with every day, family members typically are inexperienced in the medical language, tasks, principles, and procedures they are expected to do, sometimes for years to come. By figuring out why patients won't do these behaviors, AdM Coaches can modify or replace tasks and increase the likelihood of adherence.

Key points:

- AdM Home Coaching is a science-based approach to changing or adding new behaviors for healthier results.
- AdM Home Coaching relies on data and information about behavior, especially what happens before and after the action to promote healthy decisions.

- AdM Home Coaching is based on the principle that behavior is influenced by the environment and controlled precisely by the consequences of the behavior (what the patient gets out of the act).

- AdM Home Coaching looks to make meaningful changes for patients and family members (people) in order to form healthy habits.

Now It's Your Turn:

- Take the B-MAAS/B-PAAS (Appendix G & H) assessments for yourself or your patient. See if you are "At-Risk" for non-adherence.

- On a sheet of paper, write down all the tasks that your doctor has asked you to do (such as take 2 (or 15) pills twice a day, stretch leg muscles for 15 min. per day, etc.) Try to list as many things as possible. You can always add to the list later.

Behavioral Science

What do we mean by the term behavior? Behavior is defined as anything that a person does that can be observed and measured by at least one other person. A behavior is anything you see someone doing and you can measure it (how many times did it occur, how long did it happen, etc.) Examples of behaviors include talking, sitting, standing, walking, writing, waiting, rocking, reading, watching television, playing video games, and eating. (Please note this is not an all-encompassing list of behaviors).

Emily Dickinson, the 19th Century poet, stated, "Behavior is what a man does. It is not what he thinks, feels, or believes." As Adherence Management Home Coaches©, you will focus on "what people do." Cognitive behaviorists and Motivational Interviewing focus on "what people think, feel or believe." A simple description of the difference in approaches is "When I feel better, I will exercise" (Motivational) vs. "When I exercise, I feel better" (Applied behavior approach).

What Is Behavior?

On the surface, you may think this is the dumbest question in the world. Everyone knows what behavior is. After all, people have been behaving and misbehaving for thousands of years. I have sat through countless morning reports to catch up on the events of the previous day in nursing facilities and hospitals. A part of that ritual is Risk Management describing events of interest. "We had three behaviors last night," or a similar phrase is stated, and the report moves on to the next item of interest.

With several hundred patients, I should hope there were a lot more than just three behaviors. What even nurses and staff fail to realize is that all behaviors are the actions we do, not just the occasional flare-ups of bad behavior. As I reflected on Dr. Lindsley's definition: "If a dead person can do perfectly, it's not behavior." Hopefully, there were hundreds of behaviors during the previous day and evening. Even clinical professionals, with thousands of hours of experience, have difficulty understanding behavior. As you continue through this text, you will gain a better understanding of behavior and how to either increase or decrease adherent behaviors. By the way, a dead person can make no mistakes. They can appear to be in no apparent distress. They can also not renew their medications or miss the time to take a pill or check their blood sugar. Behavior is doing something that can be seen and measured by others.

There is often a common misconception, in the health services arena, that the term behavior only applies to problem behaviors like hitting, biting, punching, kicking, and slapping, eating inedible objects (pica), elopement, throwing items, and breaking things. While these are behaviors, the term behavior refers to all actions, adherent (what we want to happen again and/or more often) or non-adherent (what we want to stop or happen less often), as long as these behaviors can be observed and recorded.

Clinicians trained as AdM Coaches© work with patients and AdM Home Coaches to increase or decrease behaviors. Motivational Interviewing practitioners work to change erroneous thinking or ambivalence and then hope these changes in "wrong-thinking" are reflected by desired patient behaviors.

My Patient Had No Behaviors Today.

Dr. Ogden Lindsley stated that if a dead person can do a behavior correctly, it is not a behavior. When people first work with patients, they often report to the oncoming nurse, "John didn't have any behaviors today." This statement is supposed to inform the new nurse that John didn't have any non-adherent behaviors. If John is alive, I can assure you that he had behaviors. When the outgoing caregiver says, "John had no behaviors today," it is an inappropriate use of "shorthand." If John had adherent behaviors, these need to be recorded. What did he do? How many times? What reinforcers were used?

Is he getting better at doing the adherent behavior? Were you able to thin the reinforcement schedule? Did John need prompting to do the target behavior? This list goes on.

Many years ago, as a first year, first clinical rotation nursing student, my faculty supervisor directed that I look in on Mrs. Smith and check on her condition. Mrs. Smith was a pleasant 80 something-year-old patient. I made my observations and wrote, "Mrs. Smith is resting quietly and in no apparent distress." My faculty supervisor smiled approvingly, and I was on to the next task. Today, as both a nurse and behaviorist, I would have to question, based on my note, whether Mrs. Smith was actually alive. In fact, as Dr. Lindsley might point out, a dead person can rest quietly in bed and be in no apparent distress.

"Behavior is what a patient says or does." For the last 40 years, the tools available to improve adherence have focused on patient education, process improvement, and ensuring the health services delivery system does not fail the patient. The bottom line is adherence requires new behaviors that need to be reinforced over some time. Education fades over time, beliefs and feelings can change with new and competing information. Mark Twain defined this process well before the development of behavior science, "Habit is habit, not to be flung out the window, but to be coaxed downstairs one step at a time." Each Twain "coax" is, in essence, a reinforcer and each "step" a new behavior. Even well-established habits will fade if reinforcement is no longer available. Many pitchers and basketball players at the free-throw line use a variety of rituals before releasing the ball. As long as they are making strikes or putting the ball in the net, the rituals will continue because it is being reinforced by the positive results. This is how AdM Coaches achieve positive outcomes.

Key points:

- Behaviors are observable and measurable.
- Behaviors include all actions, both adherent behaviors and non-adherent behaviors.

- Behavior does not only refer to problem behaviors.

Now It's Your Turn:

- List four behaviors (actions) you do, or your patient does to stay healthy. Be specific. Break it down into individual action steps. (Reminder: Behavior can be seen and measured.)

How To Describe Behavior-The Do's And Don'ts?

While working with family members, an AdM Coach will discuss the behaviors necessary to accomplish the care plan with the patient, other authorized family members, and members of the Transitional Care Team, clinicians, and supervisors. When the AdM Coach talks about observed behaviors or describes the behavior, they need to be as specific as possible. Describe what happened. For example, aggressive behaviors that patients engage in may include hitting and kicking. When we describe the behavior, do not use the term "aggression. " Describe the behavior as hitting or yelling. Do not use labels for behavior. Aggressive, lazy, and non-adherent are labels and we can't fix labels.

Also, when describing behavior, do not make assumptions about emotions or feelings. The description needs to be based on actual observed behaviors and not interpretive beliefs. You can see a patient do a behavior. You cannot assess what their thoughts or emotions are. In other words, instead of Joe was sad today, use actions. Joe stayed in his bed and cried most of the day.

Looking at sports for a moment, follow-up interviews with coaches and players after a big game often show the difference between thoughts and emotions vs. actions and behaviors. The question, "Why do you think your team lost today, coach?" sometimes is answered with statements like, "I guess we didn't want it bad enough," or "Their heads were not in the game today," or "The other team was better motivated." None of these statements tell us anything about what behaviors were needed to win.

The same question could be answered with behaviors and actions, "Our defensive line needs to put more pressure on the opposing team by doing XYZ," or "Our quarterback will be throwing the ball a lot more in our next game."

Outcomes vs. Behaviors

One way to improve descriptions of behavior is to first identify the results or outcomes that clinicians and family members are looking for when the patient follows their plan of care. Once the outcomes are known, specify the behaviors necessary to achieve those outcomes. An example of medication adherence is achieving cholesterol levels that are consistently within normal limits (the result). The behavior(s) required to meet that result is taking Lipitor 10mg once a day by mouth (behavior) and increasing exercise gradually until it reaches 30 minutes per day (behavior) that produces new habits. These new habits achieve the result of cholesterol levels that are consistently within normal limits.

Key points:

Identify action behaviors that are observable and measurable and described in a manner that is:

- Factual.

- Non-interpretive.

- Without assumptions.

- Specific as possible.

Now It's Your Turn:

- List four non-behaviors (such as labels, states of being or descriptions.)

- List the actions that might be associated with the above non-behaviors.

- If a desired outcome or result is to lower your blood pressure, which behavior(s) will achieve this outcome?

   a) Reduce salt intake by removing saltshaker from the table.

   b) Take medications as prescribed.

   c) Follow an exercise program.

   d) Eat more Kentucky Fried Chicken®.

   e) a, b, & c.

   f) None of the above.

Behavior Must Be Described Without Using Labels.

You'll notice in the following paragraphs that I use some labels for behavior. The names for desired behavior, adherent behavior, non-adherent behavior and problem behavior are used to demonstrate what you do for all behaviors that fall into one of these categories. Labels are broad terms. Behaviors are specific actions.

Desired Behavior (Label)

Desired behavior is any action that a patient engages in that the AdM Coach wants to happen again or that the AdM Coach wants to happen more often. Sometimes, adherent behaviors are also referred to as compliant behaviors. But what are the behaviors within the labels of desired, adherent, or compliant?

This is the point I'm trying to make. Labels are not behaviors. There are times when adherent behaviors specific to a particular patient or family member, may not be considered adherent for another patient. The label, "Desired behavior," cannot be measured or agreed upon by several observers.

That is why, as you read this book, you will see increasingly specific terms as it relates to behavior.

Many behaviors are adherent and we want them to happen again or happen more often. Examples include, but are not limited to, more exercise, following dietary restrictions, taking medications as prescribed, following directions or completing tasks.

Key Points.

- Desired behavior is also referred to as adherent or compliant behavior.

- Desired behavior is any action that the patient does that we want to happen again or more often.

Now It's Your Turn:

- List three examples of adherent or desired behaviors and identify the actions.

- Below is a chart of Labels: What are some behaviors associated with these labels?

Labels:	Behaviors Associated with these labels
Lazy	Sits & watches TV all day
Spiteful	
Vindictive	
Angry	
Happy	

Non-Adherent Behavior

Non-adherent behaviors are any actions that patients engage in that could lead to worsening of their medical condition. Equally, it is failing to do behaviors that are helpful for their diagnosis. These behaviors may be perfectly fine under different conditions, but because the actions go against the plan of care, they are considered non-adherent. For instance, a person with chronic back pain is considered non-adherent when he engages in strenuous activities such as mowing the lawn. The lawn still needs to get mowed, just not by the patient with the bad back. As with adherent behavior, non-adherent behavior may be specific to the individual or family member.

However, some non-adherent behaviors are considered inappropriate regardless of who engages in them. Non-adherent behaviors may include, but are not limited to lying, biting, yelling, cursing, throwing objects, or incorrectly following the plan of care.

Key points:

- Non-adherent behaviors are also referred to as non-compliant behaviors or occasionally problem behaviors. Any actions that do not line up with the plan of care.

- Non-adherent behavior is any action that a patient does that we do not want to happen again or that we want to happen less often.

Now It's Your Turn:

- List four examples of how a patient might be non-adherent in following their care plan.

Why Do I Have To Know The Difference?

Being able to identify a behavior as adherent or non-adherent is an essential skill to determine how you will react to their behavior. That is, if your patient does an adherent behavior, will you respond with positive reinforcement and if they do a non-adherent behavior, will you respond with negative reinforcement, punishment or penalties, or ignore the behavior to put it on extinction. What to do when each of these types of behaviors occurs will be taught later in this book. For now, the focus is on identifying adherent and non-adherent behavior.

Why Not Use "Good" And "Bad" In Describing Behavior?

Behaviors themselves are neither good nor bad. Behavior is behavior. All behaviors, given the environment and events of the moment, can be either "good" or "bad." Some acts may be considered "good" in one culture and "bad" in another. Using certain food items as a reinforcer in one culture may be acceptable and yet thoroughly disgusting in another. Yelling and screaming, jumping up and down, and waving flags wildly are acceptable (adherent) behaviors at a sporting event or even as part of a riot. Given the same behavior in a school classroom, a courtroom, or in a church, mosque, or synagogue would be considered unacceptable, non-adherent or "bad." Hitting, biting, spitting, and kicking are behaviors that, given the right environment and conditions, are deemed appropriate (e.g., hitting an opponent in boxing, biting a hamburger, spitting out a grape seed, or kicking a soccer ball). In contrast, these same behaviors can be inappropriate if they are used to hit another person, bite a caregiver, spit in someone's face or kick another person. It might be confusing to a patient when they hear warnings like, "We don't kick or hit…" or "hitting and biting are bad," if they are playing a soccer game or biting into a piece of fried chicken.

ABC's Of Behavior

There are many ways to look at behavior. We are all experts at behaving and responding in our own environments. But we need to provide a framework of The Science of Behavior in order for the AdM Home Coach to promote healthy and productive behaviors in others.

While health providers and nurses tend to be good patient educators, the question becomes, "What happens to that information once it is given to the patient under their care, during treatments and/or after discharge?" What tools do AdM Coaches have in their arsenal to persuade those under them to perform at their best?

Understanding the Science of Behavior and applying these techniques will transform healthcare into a healthier, safer, and more cost-effective environment that we all know it can be.

While each part of this framework is a complete body of knowledge on its own, I'd like to quickly walk you through its elements, so we can have a common vocabulary.

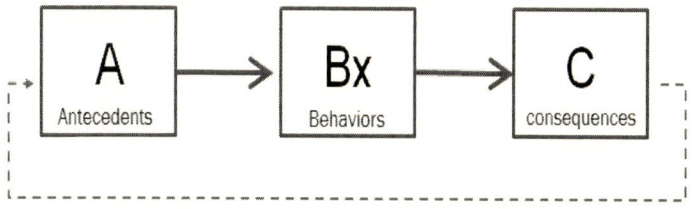

The foundation begins with the ABC Model of Behavior, which is also known as the three-term contingency – (A) Antecedent, (B) Behavior and (C) Consequence. The three-term contingency refers to the fact that every behavior (B) is influenced by an antecedent or something that comes before it to set the stage (A) and governed by what happens during or immediately after the behavior, (C) a consequence to reward or punish it.

We continuously respond to antecedents (signals, cues, roles, instructions, rules, or signs) in our internal and external environments that leads to or prompts some action (behavior). This action, in turn, leads to some result, outcome, or subsequent event happening because of that action (consequence).

ABC Behavior Chain

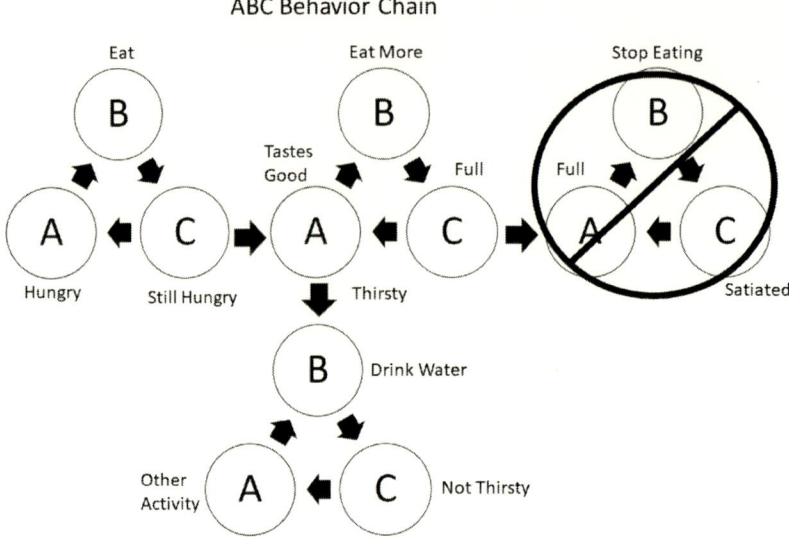

In addition, as illustrated, a consequence may then become an antecedent for another instance of the same behavior or prompt a new behavior. We have all experienced the situation where someone offers us (antecedent) chips or candy. We take one piece and eat it (behavior). It tastes good (consequence). We take another and eat it (behavior). When this is repeated many times, the behavior becomes a habit.

The ABC Model of Behavior can also become a chain of interwoven events. Consequences for one action quickly become an antecedent for another activity. This interplay happens, in real-time, within moments of one another. Consider the ABC Model of Behavior as a dynamic, fluid causal stream. Look at each part of the model as either reinforcing or triggering components and you will see that behaviors are a response to the conditions that surround them. Learn to master antecedents and consequences, and you will be able to shape the behaviors of others.

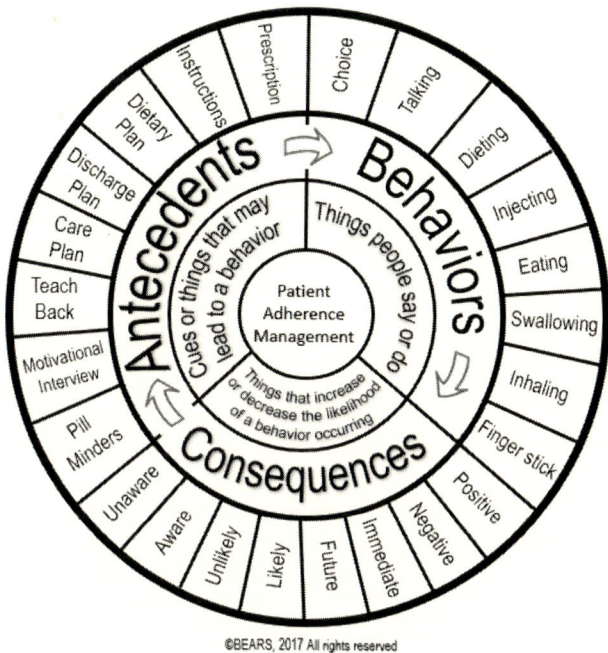

Once the ABC Model foundation is laid, a more thorough understanding of 1.) Separating actual behavior from non-behavioral descriptions; 2.) Understanding that antecedents create the environment & set the stage for action, but don't cause that behavior to happen; and, 3.) Understanding the power of consequences to either increase or decrease the occurrence of a behavior.

The circular function of the ABC Model of Behavior shows how each component is related to the others. Antecedents set the stage for adherence behaviors of following a medical care plan. Antecedents include such things as a diagnosis of a disease with prescriptions and dietary recommendations. Associated practices that are cued by these antecedents include actions like going to the pharmacy, joining a gym, and taking pills as prescribed.

How consequences are perceived by the person doing the behavior will vary from person to person. However, it is the consequences of a behavior that determine whether that behavior will increase, decrease, or stop all together. In its purest form, behaviors (B) will always have something that cues it (A) antecedent or leads to an observable action that produces some sort of result (C) consequence.

Stop signs are a cue or antecedent to stop at an intersection. It is not an action, but simply a cue for an action to occur. Care plans are a cue or antecedent for you or your patient to do the actions in the care plan. Even the disease itself is a cue or antecedent for a doctor or clinician to recommend some actions to occur to treat the illness. Without an illness to cue your behavior and unless you are going to your doctor for a wellness visit, you probably don't even think about the action of going to a doctor.

For the most part, our health is on "automatic pilot" until we have some new ache or pain. The pain serves as an antecedent for the action of making an appointment with a doctor or going to an emergency room. Without the pain, would you have planned a trip to the ER? Pain is the antecedent (A); looking for an ER, seeking inpatient care, or calling for an ambulance is the behavior (B), and the consequence is getting to the ER, receiving a diagnosis, recommendations for follow-up visits or even an admission to the hospital.

Life is an ongoing series of antecedents, behaviors, and consequences. When looking at behavior to determine how to change it, look at the ABC Model of Behavior or the antecedent, behavior, and consequence of each behavior. Looking at this information tells us why the behavior happened at that moment and whether we can expect that the behavior will occur in the future. This gives us the information we need to figure out how to get more adherent behaviors to happen and how to stop non-adherent behaviors.

AdM Home Coaches and family members are responsible for reviewing the BEARS' Adherence Consequence Analysis (BACA) completed by the transition care nurse with the patient. (See Appendix A.) This form is used to record the antecedents, behaviors, and consequences in their Adherence Improvement Plan (AIP) (See Appendix B). The BACA is extremely important in determining how effective you will be in improving adherence. Therefore, the careful and correct documentation of this data is essential. You'll be taught how to complete and monitor this form later in your training.

Remember that all behaviors, both adherent and non-adherent, have antecedents and consequences. While you may only be recording the ABCs for adherent behaviors, your ability to recognize the ABCs for both adherent and non-adherent behavior is an essential skill. You must become aware of the consequences of both to provide for your family member/patient with the appropriate reinforcement to promote healthy habits.

Key points:

- The ABCs of Behavior are Antecedent (A), Behavior (B), and Consequence (C).

- All behaviors, both adherent and non-adherent, have antecedents and consequences.

Now It's Your Turn:

- Take one behavior of your care plan and list all the antecedents and all the consequences that may occur before and after that behavior.

- Review Appendix A (BACA) and Appendix B (AIP).

Why Do We Behave?

Things people say and do (behaviors) are always a result of consequences following that behavior. People behave to get something they want or behave to avoid something they don't want. Behavior is neither right or wrong, correct or incorrect, appropriate, or inappropriate except for the environments in which they occur, and the social rules established by the societies in which they live. When we describe behavior and look at the antecedents and consequences surrounding a behavior, we are trying to figure out why a patient engaged in that behavior, at that time, and what could be reasonably predicted about that behavior in the future. By identifying this, we can put an Adherence Improvement Plan (AIP) into place to either increase adherent behavior or decrease non-adherent behavior.

"Behave" is a poorly defined label that we tell our children to do, but it doesn't convey any information about a particular action you want your children to do. It is, however, often the most straightforward term people use when talking about the actions we want people to do. To improve adherence, AdM Home Coaches need to clearly define what behavior is expected in terms of what actions your patient has to "do" to be adherent or behave.

The four most common reasons underlying all patient behavior and the purpose or reason that all patients behave as they do, is typically one of the following:

1. To get someone's attention (Attention seeking behavior).

2. To escape situations or people (Escape behavior).

3. To obtain preferred items or activities (Seeking Reinforcers).

4. To avoid a negative consequence (Avoidance behavior).

Escape or Avoidance behaviors account for many patient non-adherent behaviors. It is often the way patients communicate that the consequences of their care plan need to be changed or be modified. They're telling us that:

The plan of care is *inconvenient*.

They are *confused* about what they need to do.

Their out-of-pocket *expenses* are too high. They can't afford the medication.

Their *illness* has no symptoms, and they don't feel sick.

Forgetfulness is often a bridge excuse for one of the other seven primary consequences.

There are *side effects* they don't want to deal with.

They have *accepted* their condition and are comfortable with the outcome.

They *distrust* their clinicians or the system of care.

The BEARS mnemonic for non-adherence is ICE-IF-SAD. Greater than 90% of the reason patients choose non-adherent behaviors can be found within these eight areas of concern.

Now It's Your Turn:

- List one behavior (actions) for each of the following: Attention Seeking Behavior; Escape Behavior; Reinforcer Seeking Behavior; and, Avoidance Behavior. Be specific. Break it down into individual action steps.

- List Four Behaviors (actions) you can do, or your patient does to AVOID OR ESCAPE the healthy behaviors they know they should do. Be specific. Break it down into individual action steps they do to avoid correct behaviors.

Antecedents To Behavior.

If our goal is to change behavior, we need to identify what specific behavior we are changing. Therefore, we must describe the behavior in as much detail as possible as learned earlier. In addition, we must also look at what is going on in the environment around the patient just before the behavior happens. These are called antecedents.

Antecedents influence whether your patient knows that they must engage in a behavior at that moment. Just as with behaviors, antecedents are to be described in a factual and specific manner.

Numerous environmental events are antecedents, and in fact, almost everything in our environment influences whether we will engage in a behavior at that very moment or not. Before we look at some examples of antecedents that are often seen within our program, let's look at some examples of how antecedents influence us in our everyday lives.

Antecedent Example One: You're driving down the highway and speeding. You see a police car on the side of the road. You immediately hit the brakes to slow down.

The antecedent in this example is a police car, and the behavior is hitting the brakes to slow down. The police car is something in the environment that influenced whether you would change the speed at which you are driving (behavior). Would you slow down or hit the brakes if you did not see the police car? Probably not. The police car was the antecedent that caused you to slow down at that moment.

Antecedent Example Two: You are at home, and the phone rings. You pick up the phone and begin talking to your friend about your evening.

The antecedent is the phone ringing, and the behavior is picking up the phone and talking. The phone ringing is something in the environment that influenced you to pick up the phone. Would you think of the phone if it had not been ringing? Not unless you're going to call someone. Thus, the phone ringing (A) caused you to pick up the phone (B) at that moment.

Antecedent Example Three: You're leaving work, and it's raining outside. Before you go out, you open your umbrella.

The antecedent is the rain, and the avoidance behavior is opening your umbrella. The rain is something in the environment that you want to avoid, and it influenced or cued you to open your umbrella. Would you open your umbrella if it wasn't raining? Probably not. Thus, the rain (A) caused you to open your umbrella (B) at that moment.

As stated earlier, there are numerous antecedents; and, for almost every behavior, there are individually identifiable antecedents. Some particular cue, action, or events that typically precedes or comes before a behavior to signal a behavior to occur. Here are some typical precursors to action.

Patient Example 1: You ask a patient to take his medication, and the patient does take the meds, the antecedent is your instruction to take medicine, and the behavior is the patient taking the drug. Would this person have taken his or her medication if you had not asked him or her to? Maybe, but maybe not. Thus, your instruction to take their medication set the stage for the patient to take their meds at that moment.

Patient Example 2: Let's look at a variation of the above example. You tell a patient to wait in an Exam Room, and he/she leaves the room, what is the antecedent, and what is the behavior? The antecedent is still the instruction to wait but the behavior of leaving the room is non-adherent. Behavior may not be precisely what you are expecting. Instead, it is simply what the patient does after your instructions (the antecedent). Therefore, in this example, you might say that your direction to wait set the stage for the patient to choose to stay or leave the room at that moment.

Patient Example 3: You're about to do wound care with your patient. You get the materials needed without saying anything to the patient about it being wound care time. When you get the materials, the patient yells at you. What is the antecedent for the behavior of yelling? The antecedent is not as apparent as the previous verbal instruction, but rather it is subtler. The antecedent is you bringing in the materials necessary for the wound care, and the behavior is the "patient yelling" at you. In this example, you might say that getting the materials set the stage for this patient to yell at you at that moment.

Patient Example 4: You are assigned to a patient, and while she is sitting in her bed, you begin talking to others in the room about what you watched on television last night. The patient gets angry and verbally abuses you. What is the antecedent and behavior? The antecedent is again a little subtler than simple instruction. The antecedent is you talking to other people (i.e., Giving attention to someone other than the patient) and the behavior is the angry verbal abuse. In this example, you might say that your talking with other people prompted the patient to verbally abuse you at that moment. This antecedent brings us to an essential point about antecedents.

Antecedents, or what is happening in the environment around the patient at the time a behavior occurs, does not always have to be something added to the environment, as in an instruction. It can also be the removal of something or taking away something from the environment, as in the last example. In example four, you removed your attention, and this is what prompted the behavior to occur. The antecedent to many behaviors may be the removal of your attention either by talking to someone else or by walking away. It is imperative that patients are engaged, and caregivers are focused on them and giving them attention when we are with them. Merely interacting with patients can decrease the number of problem behaviors that are caused by an apparent lack of attention.

Patient Example 5: Just as the removal of attention can be a typical antecedent, another common antecedent is removing a leisure activity. For example, a patient is watching a favorite TV show, and you announce it's time to go to PT, and the patient gets angry and hits the caregiver. The antecedent is telling them they must leave their favorite program and the behavior is hitting in anger. Would this patient have become angry if you had waited until the end of the TV show? Probably not. Therefore, your interrupting the TV show prompted this person to get mad at that moment.

Patient Example 6: Similarly, removing food from a patient or denying a patient's request for food are two other typical antecedents. An example of denying a patient's demand for food follows. The family member is sitting down, eating his lunch when he asks for McDonald's French fries. Because you do not have McDonald's French fries and you cannot get them, you tell your family member that he or she cannot have them. The family member throws his plate across the room. What are the antecedent and the behavior? The antecedent is you denying his request for McDonald's fries, and the behavior is throwing the plate across a room. Would this family member have thrown the plate if you had not denied the fries? Maybe he would have, but at that moment, the denial prompted the behavior.

Patient Example 7: Just as the denial about food requests can be considered an antecedent, so can the denial of any other request. For example, it is raining outside, and your patient wants to go swimming. You deny this request because it is raining, and the patient yells at you. What are the antecedents, and what is the behavior? The antecedent is you denying the family member's request to go outside, and the behavior is yelling at you. Would the family member have yelled at you if you'd let him go out? Probably not. Thus, the denial prompted him to get angry and yell at that moment.

While most of the above examples describe the antecedents in terms of problem behaviors, antecedents do not just occur before problem behaviors; they occur all the time. There are antecedents for every action. Whether the behavior is adherent, and we want it to happen again or increase in frequency; or, it is non-adherent, and we want it to stop or decrease occurring, does not influence whether an antecedent is present. It is safe to assume that there is an antecedent for every behavior.

The majority of commercial solutions and devices for improving patient adherence focus on antecedents. One reason for choosing antecedents as a means for behavioral change is that most antecedents seem to be a reasonable and inexpensive way to change behavior. Pill-minders, buzzers, different colored or shaped pill bottles, reminder notes, and phone calls represent an almost endless array of devices that are all classified as antecedents. The problem with antecedents is they only set the stage for a behavior to happen, but they can be ignored or turned off. The three primary reasons for non-adherence, despite what may be written in the literature, are inconvenience, cost, and side effects. Regardless of the sophistication of the bottle, blister pack or buzzer, adherent behaviors are a function of consequences, not the antecedents that cued the behavior.

Why Focus So Much On What Happens Before The Behavior?

What happens before a behavior sets the stage for whether the behavior will occur at that moment in time. As an AdM Home Coach, it is essential to learn about antecedents for a few reasons. First, the caregiver's behaviors and actions can become antecedents to your patient's behavior. It is important to be aware of the impact that you and your activities have on your patient.

For example, if you interact with your patient, but you are in a bad mood because you got a speeding ticket on the way in to work, it might set the stage for non-adherent behavior from your patient.

Second, to change behavior, we need to know what might be causing that particular behavior to happen at that moment. Third, as an AdM Home Coach, you will be responsible for recording the antecedents for a patient's non-adherent behavior. A thorough understanding of antecedents will help you ensure that this information will be reported accurately and correctly.

Key points:

- Antecedents are things in the environment that happen just before a behavior.

- Antecedents are to be described factually.

- Antecedents are to be described as accurately as possible.

- All behaviors have an antecedent.

- Common antecedents include instructions or cues, attention from AdM Home Coaches, lack of awareness from AdM Home Coaches, removal of attention, removal of antecedent items or objects, and so forth.

Now It's Your Turn:

- List four antecedents (cues) that would come before a behavior to stay healthy.

- List one device you have or use that prompts you to do a specific behavior.

Consequences Of Behavior

When it comes to describing possible consequences of behavior, many people think "consequence" means punishment. They believe that punishment will make wrong behavior stop and replace it with right behavior. They have not discovered the power of Positive Reinforcement. Positive reinforcement rewards correct behavior and increases the likelihood of developing it into a new habit. Punishment, without correction and positive reinforcement, ensures people will develop workarounds and escape/avoidance behaviors. The consequence chart shown here is a more realistic representation of all the possible consequence outcomes.

Five Potential Types Of Consequences

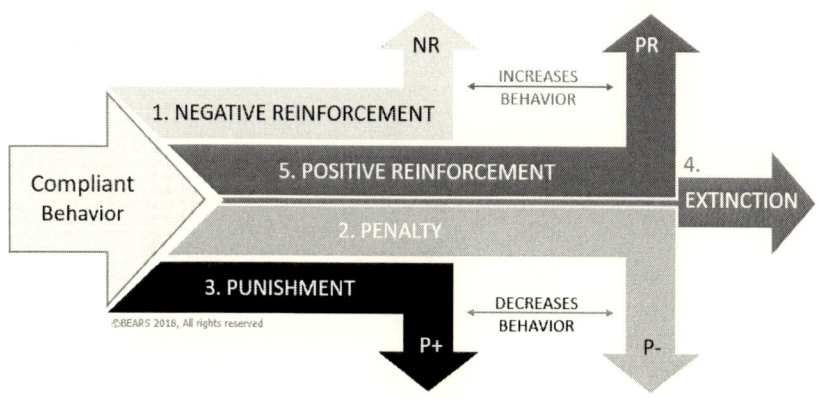

Many people gravitate to the use of negative reinforcement, followed by penalty, punishment, and extinction because of the adage they grew up with, "Do it or Else…"

The reason I listed positive reinforcement as number "5" is all too often, positive reinforcement is the "last resort" option instead of a first choice. Yet, when people are asked about their ability to influence others, they usually respond that they are very reinforcing toward others.

Consequences: What Happens After The Behavior?

We have already established the importance of behavior and antecedents in AdM Home Coaching. However, there is one more factor that influences whether the behavior will occur. These are events that happen after a behavior. What happens immediately after behaviors are called consequences. You may wonder how activities after a behavior can have an impact on future behavior.

Consequences determine whether patients will do the same behavior in the future. It shows us what patients get out of behaving that way. If they get something they like or want, they are more likely to repeat that behavior in the future. If they are punished after doing a behavior, they will be less likely to do the same behavior in the future.

As an AdM Home Coach, it is essential to learn about consequences for three reasons. First, your behavior and your actions can also serve as reinforcers to your patient's behavior, especially when you unknowingly reward certain behaviors and withhold others. It is essential to be aware of the impact that you and your actions have on family members who happen to be your patient. Second, to change behavior, you need to know what you can do to have that behavior happen more often or less frequently in the future. Third, as an AdM Home Coach, you will record the consequences for your family member/patient's behavior. A thorough understanding of consequences will help ensure that this information is recorded correctly.

Consequences influence whether the behavior will occur again in the future, while antecedents may influence or prompt whether a behavior will occur at that moment. Typically, positive consequences that patients like or want will make behaviors more likely to happen in the future, and negative consequences that patients don't like or want will make the behavior less likely to happen in the future. Just as with behaviors and antecedents, consequences must be described in a factual and specific manner.

Consequences can be used to strengthen both adherent and, unfortunately, non-adherent behaviors. Understanding consequences helps us in our effort to increase adherent behaviors. Consequences also are used in our efforts to decrease non-adherent behaviors that we do not want to see happen again or that we want to see happen less frequently.

Consequences That Decrease Behavior.

Negative reinforcement (NR, R-) is when a behavior results in avoiding an unpleasant consequence, such as wearing a jacket on a cold day. This behavior decreases the intensity of the cold weather and results in strengthening the behavior of wearing a coat. An example of negative reinforcement in healthcare may occur when we get a headache, we take an aspirin. As a result of taking aspirin (the behavior), the headache goes away (pain removal is the negative reinforcing consequence (NR, R-)), and in the future, you're more likely to take an aspirin to get rid of a headache.

NR, R- represents a two-edged sword when it comes to patients adhering to their plan of care. Although, in this case the behavior increases when avoiding unpleasant consequences. In other words, taking medications (behavior) to prevent pain (NR, R-), increases the likelihood of continuing to take medication. However, when unpleasant consequences arise from following a medication regimen, the behavior that is reinforced is to avoid the penalties and punishers of adherence (i.e., inconvenience, side-effects, expense, etc.) The negative aspects of following the care plan will cause non-adherence (avoidance) behaviors to increase.

Punishment And Penalty

Punishment and Penalty are two concepts that might seem on the surface to be inappropriate in the delivery of health services. Most of us associate punishment as a "consequence" for having done an illegal behavior, getting caught, and then "getting something we don't want."

Punishment is rarely the starting place for clinicians in their plan of care. At least, that's what they believe from the clinician's perspective. The definition of Punishment is any situation in which the consequence of a behavior produces a negative or unpleasant result, and behavior decreases. The primary function of completing a BEARS Adherence Consequence Analysis (See Appendix A – BACA) is discovering punishers that are embedded in a patient's discharge plan or care plan. The easiest way to decide if a care plan is punishing is to look at the consequences. If adherent behavior is not occurring, then punishers are present. Keep in mind that what might be punishing for one person may be reinforcing for another.

The most common punishers affecting a patient's choice to follow a particular plan of care (a behavior) are inconvenience, expense, and side effects (consequences). Normal people avoid punishment and quickly stop doing behaviors that result in negative consequences. The key element of doing a BACA is to look at the consequences of a care plan, from the patient's perspective.

Given a correct diagnosis and an appropriate plan for disease management is likely to have a positive outcome from the clinician's perspective. However, it is the patient who must take the prescriptions, have dietary restrictions, exercise mandates, and various other demands at home when they are discharged. One of the roles for AdM Home Coaches is to see where these problem areas arise to see if they can be mitigated before discharge, or adherence behaviors positively reinforced to overcome the negative aspects of treatment.

Another consequence that has an impact on adherence is the often-used warnings from staff members and others that may sound like, "If you don't take your medications, you could die." Another popular phrase is, "Do you want to have a stroke (heart attack, asthma attack, develop cancer, etc.)?"

On face value alone, these comments provide very little help in producing adherent behaviors and yet family and friends, as well as providers and clinicians, often toss these statements out, hoping to scare their patients into new habits.

Punishment and penalties did not work in the Garden of Eden, "If you eat of the fruit from the tree of the knowledge of Good and Evil, you shall surely die," and it is equally ineffective as a behavioral change tool today. That fact that neither Adam nor Eve immediately died from eating the "apple" from their perspective, and they perceived a positive reward of having their understanding enlightened is the very definition of non-adherence.

An In-Depth Look At Consequences.

Based on a case study published by Dr. Michael Stein entitled "*Losing Control*"[1], we look at how consequences can impact adherence. Dr. Stein's brilliantly written article describes his clinical relationship with a patient named Beatriz and her struggle with HIV/AIDS and its various treatments. Using the tools and knowledge he had available at the time, before AdM Coaching, he focused on several approaches to try to increase her adherence, to no avail.

In Appendix C1, we filled out a BACA example showing how consequences could be analyzed to determine the contributing factors of Beatriz's non-adherence. There were several other approaches that Dr. Stein might have used. I have written an in-depth analysis of Dr. Stein's dilemma using all our tools and techniques. Several recommendations are described in Appendix D.

---

1 Stein, Michael, (2016) Losing Control, Harvard Review. Accessed online https://www.harvardreview. org/content/losing-control/. The author highly recommends reading Dr. Stein's article. Non-adherence affects everyone. Dr. Stein reveals the frustration physicians also face with their non-adherent patients.

Consequences That Increase Behavior.

While punishers and penalties decrease the likelihood that a behavior will occur again, one specific type of consequence increases behavior, Positive Reinforcement (R+). It is essential for all AdM Coaches to understand, for behaviors to increase, they must use reinforcers.

To reinforce something means to strengthen or increase it. Reinforcement is a consequence AdM Coaches use to strengthen or improve behaviors so they will be more likely to happen again or will occur more often in the future.

There are two types of reinforcement, Positive Reinforcement (R+) and Negative Reinforcement (R-), which we discussed earlier. Positive reinforcement (R+) is when a behavior is followed by something that the patient wants or needs that results in strengthening that behavior.

In the wound care example previously mentioned, if the patient received praise R+ (great job with your wound care today!) for completing the wound care treatment, would he be more likely or less likely to complain about wound care in the future? He would be less likely to complain and more likely to complete the wound care because the behavior (completing the treatment) was followed by the consequence of positive reinforcement R+ (great job! You did that treatment well.) If he had completed the wound care and had not been given positive reinforcement, the behavior may or may not be as successful, and the yelling might continue.

In the jacket example previously mentioned, you wear a jacket to avoid getting cold (NR (R-)). In the future, you are more likely to wear a coat on cold days. You're more likely to use a coat (behavior) in the future because it was successful at avoiding cold (R-) in the past.

Increasing And Decreasing Behavior

Taking medications on time and increasing persistence to the end of creating new habits will require an increase in positive reinforcement (R+) at every opportunity. As habits are developed, reinforcement can be thinned. Keep in mind that reinforcement should never be abandoned. Remind patients why they are being reinforced from time to time. Look at ways to decrease inconvenience and expenses. When side effects are present, look for additional ways to reduce the impact of side effects.

Key points:

- Punishment can readily be found in discharge plans.
- Punishment is in the eye of the beholder. Clinical requirements need to be evaluated through the patient's perspective.
- Threats of bad things to come to encourage patients to do something that is punishing today will seldom lead to behavior change.

Now It's Your Turn:

- List two punishing things that happen when you do, or your patient does a behavior (action) to stay healthy. Be specific. How does it make you feel?
- List two positive things that happen when you do, or your patient does a behavior (action) to stay healthy. Be specific. How does that make you feel?

What Is The Difference Between R- And P-?

Many people are confused with the term Negative Reinforcement (R-) and see it as a step in the direction of Punishers P (+) and Penalties P (-). The "R" means it is a reinforcing factor that points toward increasing behaviors, while the "P" is a punishing factor, which significantly decreases or stops behaviors. With R (-), patients "choose" to be adherent to avoid the punishing aspects of the disease process. Concurrently, patients may "choose" to be non-adherent because the "punishing aspects" of following their care plan are sufficiently stronger than any "reinforcing aspects," and any clinically adherent behavior will stop.

Negative Reinforcement, R (-) increases behavior. Avoiding being cold by wearing a jacket increases the use of putting on a coat when the environment is cold. When the environment is hot, there is little or no consideration of wearing a coat. There is nothing in the atmosphere to cue jacket-wearing behavior. Negative reinforcement (cold) increases behavior (wearing a coat) by avoiding the "potential" of discomfort, inconvenience, or loss.

Punishers (P+) decrease behavior by adding some negative consequences after a behavior occurs, making that behavior less likely to happen again.

Most long-term medications are taken to avoid some effects of a disease that may happen months or years in the future. In other words, taking drugs can be a negative reinforcer (R-) to avoid disease symptoms down the road. However, problems arise with the persistence of taking those meds if the continued appropriate use of medications has any punishing side-effects or inconveniences. Then, the punishers (P+) of receiving the pills will override any negative reinforcers (R-), and patients will stop taking their meds. Furthermore, if adherence to a medication plan does have the presence of punishers (P+) and there is no perception of what is being avoided (i.e., the patient is not aware of the benefit of taking the meds to avoid some aspect of the disease in the future), this will lead to the extinction of that behavior. This is discussed further in the section on "Extinction."

Penalties P (-) are the actual loss of something a patient already has or wants and taking that something away decreases the likelihood of that behavior happening in the future. A good example might be telling your teenager that staying out past 10 pm will result in losing the privilege of going out at all for one week. Telling a patient that if they don't follow their plan of care, it will result in being dropped from the practice. This is a form of penalty (P-) consequence.

The clinician who uses this type of penalty (P-) consequence hopes that the patient will follow their plan of care (increase behavior) to avoid losing their clinician. What the clinician doesn't realize is that punishers and penalties decrease behavior; they do not increase them. Dropping patients from their practice is the penalty (P-) for continued non-adherence. In other words, they are penalizing a non-behavior (not following doctor's orders). These types of threats will always be ineffective in changing behavior, and penalties (P-) will be invoked. Losing a non-adherent patient may be beneficial to the doctor, but it doesn't help the patient at all.

Historically, more than half of patients will stop following their care plans to avoid the perceived punishing or penalizing consequences. This avoidance behavior increases non-adherence. Clinicians, as they prepare their care plans, need to evaluate the outcomes from the patient's perspective to determine the punishers in the plan.

Key points:

- Negative reinforcement (R-) increases adherent behavior as patients attempt to avoid potential discomfort in the future (e.g., taking meds to prevent a future heart attack).

- Punishers (P+) decrease behavior because patients do not want the added punishment. The behavior will reduce or stop.

- Penalty (P-) decreases behavior because the patient knows that by doing the behavior would result in something being taken away or removed that they have or want. These are usually used to get the patient's attention quickly.

- Punishing consequences can lead to non-adherence as patients identify immediate negative aspects of their care plan they want to avoid.

Extinction

Extinction is a consequence to decrease behavior over time. Extinction occurs when there is no reinforcement or awareness of any positive consequence, and as a result, the behavior decreases and eventually stops. When a child throws a tantrum to get attention or to get something, and the child accomplishes getting that something, then the tantrum behavior is reinforced. However, if the tantrum (behavior) is completely ignored, then it is not reinforced and will eventually stop. (Be aware of the reinforcers that may also come from unlikely sources. The other customers in the store who stare and whisper about what a horrible parent you are for ignoring your child, are actually reinforcing that child's tantrum behavior, adding fuel to the fire. Parenting is not for the faint at heart.)

So, extinction is also true for people trying to follow their plan of care, but they don't perceive any apparent benefits from following the plan, nor do they get any positive feedback from their doctor or caregiver. This will result in their behavior of following the plan being put on extinction and they will likely stop adherent behaviors.

Three elements of extinction occur with patients and adherence to their plan of care.

Medication Extinction – With this extinction process, patients take their medication as prescribed but don't feel any better or worse. Their perception is the medicine is not working, so why take it?

Doctor Extinction – Patients see their provider on an infrequent basis. Often, office visits are late, and there is an extended wait time in the reception area. "If my illness was that bad, wouldn't my doctor be more concerned?"

Clinical Extinction – Clinical extinction is like a maintenance warning light on your car. "The light is on, but my car seems to be working fine. I'll take it in if I start to hear something." In many disease processes, the consequences are years away.

One of the fundamental laws of behavior is, "Behavior goes where reinforcement flows." Let's look at some examples:

Consequence Example 1: Henry is a patient and uses a rescue inhaler. He recently had an asthma attack and used his inhaler. Within a minute or two, his airway was clear, and he was breathing normally. The consequence of using the inhaler was positive and immediate. It reinforced the behavior, and Henry always keeps his inhaler in his pocket.

Consequence Example 2: Henry also has high blood pressure and stopped taking his medication. When asked why, he said he didn't notice any difference when he took it. While the drug was working, there was nothing to indicate that the cost, inconvenience, and side effects were worth it. In short, there was no reinforcement. The effectiveness of the medication was put on extinction because there was nothing positive or immediate that could reinforce his behavior. Everything associated with taking this medication was punishing. Even if cost, convenience and side-effects were not an issue, the benefit was not apparent.

AdM Home Coaches must be aware that many long-term medications are only effective over time and that reinforcement should center on adherent behavior (e.g., taking pills as prescribed) and celebrations should be scheduled when lab benchmarks or results are showing improvement. Extinction is a significant concern when it comes to non-adherence. This reality has to be considered in completing the AIP with patients.

Key points:

- Extinction decreases behavior over time.
- Extinction is when reinforcers are 1) no longer given, 2) taken away, or 3) not perceived; and, as a result, the behavior decreases and eventually stops over time.
- If medication adherent behavior is reinforced, it will likely continue.

- If medication adherent behavior is ignored, it will likely go on to extinction.

BEARS Adherence Consequence Analysis (BACA).

Over the past several years, medical and nursing literature has focused on a "patient-centered" approach to achieving improved healthcare outcomes. Historically, health services were offered in a "paternalistic" manner. This approach focused on the belief that "doctors know best." It failed to recognize that patients and their families have a say in the outcome. Patients always have a choice to accept and follow their doctor's recommendations or not. As you read more of this book, you will see references to the BEARS Adherence Consequence Analysis or BACA. This analysis is generally completed under the supervision of a Registered Nurse Adherence Management Coach and his/her patient. The results are then shared with the primary physician.

The BACA is an adaptation of Dr. Aubrey Daniel's highly regarded Performance Management PICNIC Analysis®. In Dr. Daniel's tool, for every behavior there is at least one consequence that happens as a result of that behavior. Each consequence has three pairs of characteristics that describe it. The first characteristic pair is whether the consequence is positive or negative. The second pair deals with timing. When does the consequence happen -- immediately after the behavior or sometime in the future? The third characteristic pair determines the certainty of the consequence occurring. Will the consequence always occur after the behavior or does it only occur occasionally or sometimes not at all?

There are two key differences between the PICNIC Analysis® and the BACA. First, in medicine, certainty is never a given. A treatment may likely fix an illness, but many variables determine its actual effectiveness. For this reason, we modified the third characteristic from certain and uncertain to likely and unlikely. It is likely that taking blood pressure medication will lower your blood pressure, but it is not certain, especially if you continue to eat potato chips, salted peanuts and salted pretzels every day. If medication is taken correctly, achieving improved health is "Likely," but not certain. Eating salted peanuts and pretzels would typically lead to being "Unlikely" to achieve health, however, you might still get better on your own.

The second difference is the addition of a fourth characteristic pair called perception. Is the patient aware of the consequence or not aware? Can the consequence be felt or perceived by the patient or is the consequence outside the patient's conscious awareness? Again, in medicine, we may have a disease but are unaware of its damaging effects. Or, we may take medications for a disease that has no outward symptoms. Because we are not aware that a medication is working, we don't feel any better or worse, we might stop taking it.

A consequence is any event, following a behavior, which increases or decreases the likelihood of that behavior occurring again. Consequences always contribute to the success or failure of a plan of care because while the clinical outcomes may be good for the patient from a medical perspective, these same consequences may be negative, uncertain, punishing, or even unaware to the patient from his or her perspective. Also, positive consequences that are not perceived by a patient can lead them to abandon their plan of care believing that it is not working.

Clinicians tend to look at consequences merely as the outcomes of following their treatment and "getting better" or "free from symptoms." Patients are more likely to consider consequences as personal. How will this affect me right now in terms of cost, side effects, convenience, complexity, and so on. As AdM Coaches review the consequences from the patient's perspective, the patient and coach will gain added insights into how the doctor might need to modify the care plan to increase opportunities for adherence.

A Brief Look At How To Use BACA.

Learning to look at consequences from the patient's perspective is a point of view that is often overlooked. The BACA provides a platform for looking at the Antecedent-Behavior-Consequence model from the patient's eyes. First, we identify the things (Antecedents) that may cue or prompt a patient's behavior. In this portion of the BACA, we use the prompt, "This got me thinking…" or "When I am …, I do this behavior," to identify antecedents. The antecedent for going to a doctor could be abdominal pain or any other symptom. Many symptoms may not rise to an action level. In this case, it may be a verbal cue from a spouse or significant other that serves as the antecedent. Antecedents are any cue that may lead to a behavior. Antecedent: I have a symptom. This leads to a Behavior: Making a phone call. The Consequence: An appointment is made with a doctor or clinic.

There is a whole series of Antecedent-Behavior-Consequence loops that happen in healthcare. We call these behavior chains. You, being in the exam room, cues the behavior of an examination by the physician that leads to the consequence of a diagnosis. The diagnosis is a cue for a plan of care. The plan of care includes a prescription. All of these cues should lead to behaviors that support the plan. The behaviors can include taking medications by mouth, one or more times a day. Going to the pharmacy to pick up a prescription is a behavior. Paying for the prescription is a behavior. There are numerous ABC loops in the healthcare behavior chain. Whether any particular behavior is repeated enough times to form a habit within this chain will depend on the consequence that behavior receives.

As AdM Coaches sit with patients to do their BEARS Adherence Consequence Analysis™ (BACA), it is important in the next section to pinpoint the specific behavior that needs to be changed or the new habit that needs to be developed. Too many patients abandon their plan of care or their medication regimes within days or weeks of discharge because specific behaviors were not part of the implementation plan. While the goal is always 100% adherence, in many instances, an 85% medication compliance rate might be sufficient to maintain therapeutic levels. It might be appropriate to set a starting goal of 85% adherence as the planned intervention and reinforce adherence up to 100% until the new habit is formed.

Keep in mind, there are medications that require 100% adherence to prevent unwanted clinical outcomes. These should be identified for patients and appropriate education provided. The information provided here does not endorse partial adherence or so called "drug holidays." We accept the reality that all human behavior that is not reinforced will return to baseline. The baseline as it relates to taking a handful of pills several times a day, is taking no pills at all. A prescription in hand and an adherence prayer by a clinician have not significantly changed patient behaviors over the last several thousand years.

During the initial patient interview, it is essential to find the consequences that may contribute to non-adherence. Keep in mind that some of the results may be unrelated on the surface. Taking a closer look at Dr. Stein's patient Beatriz, her spouse nagged her when she did not take her medications. The consequence of nagging did little to reinforce Beatriz's behavior. Some people might see this nagging behavior as good if the spouse is attention-seeking. But many of Beatriz's behaviors and excuses make no sense to someone looking in from the outside. What is important in a consequence analysis is that it makes sense to her. Although her behaviors are harming her in the long term, most of her behaviors have self-reinforcing consequences.

Numerous factors can come together to discourage taking medications. Each of these factors need to be taken into consideration as the BACA is completed. The purpose of the BACA is to identify the parts of the discharge or care plan that may lead to non-adherence. Where possible, your RN AdM Coach can have a discussion with the physician to see if some reasonable accommodations can be reached. We believe that the BACA is a patient-centered approach to achieving buy-in for the life-style changes that may be needed to support the care plan. Knowing where patients may stumble because of consequences is an important step to building a better plan. Consequences Matter™.

Consequences Are Described Using A Variety Of Terms.

Let's take a closer look at how consequences are divided into these four characteristic category pairs. The first category is Outcome Type. An Outcome Type can be either reinforcing (Positive) or punishing (Negative). The reinforcing or punishing characteristics of a consequence must always be evaluated from the patient's perspective, not necessarily the clinical result.

"Positive" means the outcome of the consequence is *rewarding* to the person who does the behavior. If a consequence is Positive, it means it strengthens the likelihood that the behavior will happen again. If a baseball player hits a home run on his first pitch, he is likely to do all the same behaviors the next time at bat. If he hits another home run, those behaviors will be strengthened. If those behaviors consistently produce the consequence of home runs (Positive) from the player's perspective, those behaviors will form into habit. When talking about Positive consequences, we could also use similar terms to describe it: *"Is the consequence satisfying?"* or *"Is the consequence constructive?"*

Consequences that are punishing, painful, unpleasant, or inconvenient to the person doing the behavior are said to be "Negative" consequences. Negative consequences might be considered *"bad"* by the patient. However, it simply describes what effect the consequence has on the behavior. "Negative" means the outcome of the consequence is punishing to the person doing the behavior, thereby weakening the likelihood that the behavior will happen again. Does the consequence reward the behavior, from the patient's perspective? Does the consequence punish the behavior, from the patient's perspective? The bottom line is this, if a person does this behavior, will the consequence outcome be "good" for them or "bad" for them? People do not routinely do behaviors when the consequence that follows is negative, punishing, painful, or unpleasant.

The second characteristic category pair looks at the effect of the *timing* of the consequence following a behavior. Consequences that are *immediate* (occur during the behavior or very shortly thereafter) are more powerful than consequences that occur at a much later time in the future. Some medications, such as rescue inhalers, have an immediate consequence. When a patient cannot breathe because of asthma or COPD, the action of using a rescue inhaler brings immediate relief. Blood pressure medications, and many other commonly used medications to treat chronic conditions, may be effective treatments but the positive consequence may be delayed for months or years into the future. An immediate consequence will strengthen a behavior much more than a future consequence.

The third characteristic category pair of the BACA examines the *likelihood or probability* that the consequence will occur. If a consequence is certain to occur every time a behavior happens, it will strengthen that behavior. If the occurrence of the consequence is uncertain (that is, you can't predict whether or not the consequence will occur), it will have the effect of weakening that behavior. As mentioned previously, we made a modification to the PICNIC Analysis® by changing the probability from *"certain" to "likely"* because in medicine, nothing is certain.

When it comes to many treatment plans or medications, while the likelihood of its effectiveness is often very high, there is always a risk when providers assure patients that clinical results are *"certain."* Clinical results are *"likely"* to occur if a target behavior of following the plan of care is carried out as prescribed, but not guaranteed. Clinical results may or may not, or *"unlikely"* to happen if a lesser behavior is done. An example of this might be choosing to eat unsalted crackers, instead of potato chips and salted pretzels to treat your high blood pressure. It is unlikely that this simple behavior will produce the clinical results you seek, but the possibility exists. Nothing in healthcare is certain or uncertain. Likely and unlikely better describe the realms of possibilities in medicine.

The fourth and final characteristic category pair of the BACA is Perception. Many effects of medical treatments may be *beneath a patient's level of perception*. The benefit of the consequence of a behavior may not be perceived by the patient, which weakens the behavior from happening again. This is radically different from Performance Management (and the PICNIC Analysis® of Dr. Daniels), where productivity in an office is simply measured by the performance of behaviors. More or less behaviors directly result in more or less productivity. In medicine, behaviors and clinical results are reinforced and measured separately. Measuring and reinforcing the behavior of taking a blood sugar pill every day is separated from the lab blood test measuring a patient's A1C levels. That reality led us to add this fourth consequence criteria, *PERCEPTION*.

Many patients become non-adherent with their treatment behaviors stating, *"I didn't feel the medication was working, so I stopped taking it!"* Being aware that a consequence is present and working will strengthen the behavior to continue or increase in the future. Not being aware that the consequence is present and working will weaken the behavior as if the consequence wasn't even there.

Four Consequence Characteristic Category Pairs

The following table summarizes the Four Consequence Characteristic Pairs and provides alternative words to describe each characteristic to assist in filling out the BACA.

BEARS' Consequence Categories

Outcome		Timeliness	
Positive (P)	**Negative (N)**	**Immediate (I)**	**Future (F)**
Good	Bad	Now	Later
Satisfying	Annoying	During	After
Advantageous	Disadvantageous	Direct	Indirect
Convinced	Unconvinced	Close	Distant
Confident	Unconfident	Proximate	Ultimate
Constructive	Destructive		

Likelihood		Perception	
Likely (L)	**Unlikely (U)**	**Aware (A)**	**Not aware (N)**
Sure	Unsure	Perceived	Unperceived
Certain	Uncertain	Know	Don't know
Reliable	Unreliable	Mindful	Unmindful
Dependable	Undependable	Obvious	Oblivious
No doubt	Doubtful		
Unambiguous	Ambiguous		

The Complete Consequence Picture.

Every consequence is designated with all four characteristics. A consequence that is Positive/Immediate/Likely/Aware (PILA) is good and rewarding for the patient (Positive), occurs during or immediately after the behavior (Immediate), has a high probability of always occurring after the behavior (Likely), and the patient perceives that the consequence is present and working (Aware). These types of consequences will be highly effective at getting the behavior that it is associated with, to occur again. A consequence that is Negative/Immediate/Likely/Aware (NILA) is just as powerful, but it will cause the behavior to decrease or stop. These consequences are painful or bad for the person (Negative), occurs during or immediately after the behavior (Immediate), has a high probability of always occurring after the behavior (Likely), and the patient perceives that the consequence is present and working (Aware). NILA consequences will severely weaken a behavior's strength to continue again. An example of a NILA consequences are medication side effects that do not diminish over time or the high cost of medications that takes a big chunk out of a patient's budget. If a patient experiences a painful, immediate reaction every time they take a medication, they will seek ways to avoid the NILA consequence, even if that includes stopping the behavior of taking the medication.

Strength Of A Consequence.

Health related consequences present a wide range of strengths as they relate to human behaviors. Medication behaviors may have consequences that are POSITIVE, but FUTURE, UNLIKELY (meaning you don't know if they will work or not), and NOT AWARE that the medication is working (PFUN) (e.g., lowering blood pressure, managing A1C results, keeping viral loads low, etc.), while the consequences of cost, side effects and inconvenience of the medications tend to be *NEGATIVE, IMMEDIATE, LIKELY, and the patient is very AWARE (NILA)*. You can rest assured that the power of a NILA will defeat most POSITIVE, FUTURE, UNLIKELY, NOT AWARE (PFUN) consequences every time unless an additional reinforcer is added to the equation.

Because clinical outcomes extend well beyond the behavior of taking a pill, they tend to be ineffective at influencing the behavior itself. These clinical results tend to be POSITIVE, *FUTURE*, LIKELY, but NOT AWARE (at least until lab test are done in the future). These PFLN consequences may be good at addressing and treating a disease, but are useless in reinforcing the behaviors necessary for getting the medication into the patient in the first place. Managing an acute infection with antibiotics represent a PFLA outcome. It is a little stronger in influencing the behavior of pill-taking than a PFLN or a PFUN because the patient is aware that the medication is working in a relatively short amount of time. The pill-taking behavior may still need an additional reinforcer consequence, but the PFLA will strengthen the behavior as well. Long-term medications for chronic diseases like hypertension or hyperlipidemia or HIV/AIDS, etc. may represent a PFLN consequence for managing the disease, but represent NILA consequence, from the patient's perspective, in terms of long-term costs, side effects and inconveniences, while the desired clinical outcome may be years away.

As the RN AdM Coach fills out the BACA and goes over the various consequences with the patient, they should consider using many of the similar words or synonyms in the same category. This will help the patient understand how the consequence affects them, from their perspective. Patients may have a hard time thinking in terms of positive or negative but might identify with "good and rewarding" or "bad and punishing." Be familiar with the synonyms so you can help your patient or family member who might have a difficult time understanding how to describe a particular consequence.

To Do or Not To Do.

The BACA is divided into many sections. Columns are arranged for Antecedents, Behaviors, and Consequences. The consequence section is further divided into the characteristic pairs for each consequence. Once analyzed, each consequence is identified as one that strengthens or one that weakens the behavior in question.

The analysis is further divided into behaviors that don't follow the plan of care and behaviors that do follow (with all the antecedents and consequences associated with those behaviors.) Each behavior should be addressed with the patient one-at-a-time. Review with the patient all the consequences when they "Don't Follow" their care plan. Then repeat the process for when they "Do Follow" their care plan. This will become clearer as you look at the BACA, as well as the one we completed on Beatriz.

BEARS Targeted Consequence Analysis of Patient Care Plan

	Patient:			Behavior Outcome							
	Date:			Clinician							
	AdM Coach:										

	ANTECEDENTS	BEHAVIOR	CONSEQUENCES	P	N	I	F	L	U	A	N
	"These got me thinking"	"If I did this…"	"These things could happen…"								
1											
2											
3											
4											
5											
6		What may happen if I									
7		DON'T FOLLOW the									
8		Target Behavior									
9		described above?									
10											
11											
12											
13											
14											
			TOTAL	0	0	0	0	0	0	0	0

	ANTECEDENTS	BEHAVIOR	CONSEQUENCES	P	N	I	F	L	U	A	N
	"These got me thinking"	"If I did this…"	"These things could happen…"								
1											
2											
3											
4											
5											
6		What may happen if I									
7		FOLLOW the Target									
8		Behavior described									
9		above?									
10											
11											
12											
13											
14											
			TOTAL	0	0	0	0	0	0	0	0

	PILA	NILA	PIUA	NIUA	PFLA	NFLA	PFUA	NFUA	PILN	NILN	PIUN	NIUN	PFLN	NFLN	PFUN	NFUN	Total
	Most power		Middle power		Middle power		Least power		Least weakness		Middle weakness		Middle weakness		Most weakness		
Nonadherent																	0
Adherent																	0
Difference																	0

Patient Centered Means Looking At Consequences From The Patient's Perspective.

The BACA allows AdM Coaches and patients to look at the consequences of following their plan of care and not following it. It also provides a clear indication of areas where the AdM Coach may be able to modify the plan to meet a patient's needs (Patient Centered). This will increase the likelihood the patient will follow the plan. Patient education creates short-term knowledge and some understanding of "what" needs to be done. Consequence analysis tells clinicians and clients what may likely happen when they choose to follow or not to follow their plan of care.

This consequence analysis information is critical when developing a BEARS Adherence Improvement Plan (AIP) for each "at-risk" patient. The BACA is best completed in a conversational manner and without judging any of the patient's answers. Many of the techniques used in "Motivational Interviewing" can be used as an approach to fact gathering for the BACA.

When it comes to filling out a BEARS Adherence Improvement Plan (AIP), knowledge of the consequences of being Not Aware of symptoms or the lack of perceived improvements after treatment *must be considered* to ensure adherent behaviors are properly reinforced.

Determine The Behaviors You Need For Success.

Just as with any diagnosis, knowing the problem is essential in developing a plan to manage adherent and non-adherent behaviors. There are many consequences related to following a plan of care that must be analyzed, *from the patient's perspective*. Far too often, health services assume that treatment recommendations make perfect sense to patients. But, for more than half of the patient population, the opposite is true. Once health services has determined that a patient is "at-risk" for non-adherence, they can use the BACA to look at the "Target" behavior and all the consequences associated with doing it or not.

What May Happen If...

"Behavior is what a person does. It is not what s/he thinks, feels or believes." With that clear definition, the behavior Beatriz needs to do every day, is to take her Prescobix, by mouth, one time daily.

With each requirement in a care plan, it is important to identify the consequences if patients follow their care plan and if they choose to not follow it. There are advantages in each direction. Ideally, patients will choose to be adherent. Understanding what happens to patients who fail to follow their plan of care is necessary information for them to maintain their choice of adherence. A patient centered approach focuses on the patient expressing their understanding of the consequences of choosing not to follow the care plan and creating a list of all possible consequences, both for and against.

Evaluating whether the consequences are positive or negative will come later. Right now, we are simply creating the list of all possible consequences.

Avoid going back and forth between "don't follow" and "follow." It may be confusing to both the AdM Coach© and the patient if suddenly either party goes back to "don't follow." If the patient suddenly thinks of several "don't follow" consequences, stop for a minute and make sure they understand you are again looking at the consequences of not following the care plan and write them down. Then go back to the consequences for "following" and ensure they understand you are now looking for what might happen if they take their medication(s) as prescribed.

Dr. Stein thought it was important for Beatriz to get some help from a counselor and to share information about her disease with her family. In the article, she was adamant about not talking with anyone else. A BACA evaluation offers some background as to why she felt so strongly about this recommendation. We'll explore this a little later.

Antecedents In The BACA.

By the time a patient is completing a BEARS Adherence Consequence Analysis© (BACA), many things have happened that led to this moment. The antecedents should be written down and can be a combination of symptoms, advice from friends and family, or other cues that medical help is needed. By definition, antecedents are anything that prompts or leads a person to an action or behavior. Antecedents are important to identify in the BACA as they may point to other behaviors that may strengthen or weaken target behaviors that will be necessary for adherence. It is important to list as many events as possible that are associated with leading up to the behavior being studied. Keep in mind, antecedents don't have to match consequences one for one. Some antecedents may serve as a reinforcer for behavior as you will see later in Dr. Stein's text. (Spouse nagging can be a positive reinforcer. Even though it seems like it would be a punisher, for people who need attention, bad attention is better than no attention at all.)

The antecedents for Beatriz are highlighted on the left side of her BACA. You will find the antecedents are the same for doing and not doing the Target Behavior (Take Prescobix 1 time daily). Recall that antecedents can be any cue or prompt that could result in the target behavior. The essential word is "could." Antecedents do no increase the likelihood that a behavior will occur. It simply sets the stage for the behavior to occur. A diagnosis of HIV is an antecedent for Dr. Stein to write a prescription for Beatriz. The diagnosis and written prescription are antecedents for Beatriz to purchase the prescription. The antecedent for Dr. Stein is significantly more compelling than it is for Beatriz. The consequences for Dr. Stein (e.g., malpractice) can be more quickly punishing than for Beatriz. Just remember, the BACA is always filled out from the patient's point of view, not the health service provider.

Antecedents can be a chain of events that may have begun with Beatriz not feeling well when this episode began three years earlier. She was seen by another physician who diagnosed her with HIV. Some of the antecedents may be more compelling than others. For example, approaching a stop sign while driving a car is likely to be more compelling than it is for the passenger. It changes the driver's behavior while the passenger's behavior is unchanged. If it appears the driver is not paying attention and is approaching the stop sign at a high speed, it is likely the passenger's behavior will change quickly.

Antecedents help patients to understand how they arrived at this point where a change in behavior is needed. It also points out other potential consequences that patients may want to avoid. Consequences, such as "spouse nagging," can become antecedents to following the care plan to avoid getting something you don't want (e.g., nagging.)

Disease symptoms can be an antecedent if they are perceived. Too often, the lack of symptoms support the belief that nothing bad is going to happen and patients decide taking their medications are a waste of time. Antecedents need to be explored with patients to see which antecedents may be more useful in changing behavior.

BEARS Targeted Consequence Analysis for Plan of Care

Patient Name	Beatriz		Target Behavior:	Take Prescobix 1 time daily
Date:	06/11/2016	Provider prescribing plan of care	Dr. Stein	
AdM Coach©	R. Wright, PhD, RN			

Plan of Care/HIV diagnosis

ANTECEDENTS	BEHAVIOR	CONSEQUENCES	P	N	I	F	L	U	A	N
Diagnosed with HIV Fear of death Family worried Fear of lost work Fear of disability May lose job	What may happen if I *don't follow* the Target Behavior described above?									

ANTECEDENTS	BEHAVIOR	CONSEQUENCES	P	N	I	F	L	U	A	N
Visit to Drs. Office Diagnosis Prescription Teachback Counseling Disease symptoms Spouse nagging	What may happen if I *follow* the Target Behavior described above?									

ANTECEDENTS	BEHAVIOR	CONSEQUENCES	P	N	I	F	L	U	A	N
Fear of the unknown Beliefs	Disclose illness and seek counseling									

		Strongest to Weakest Consequences								Extinction Consequences							
⟶ Consequence		PILA	NILA	PIUA	NIUA	PFLA	NFLA	PFUA	NFUA	PILN	NILN	PIUN	NIUN	PFLN	NFLN	PFUN	NFUN
		Most Power		Upper Middle		Lower Middle		Least Power		Least Weakness		Upper Middle		Lower Middle		Most Weakness	
Behavior(s)																	

List All The Consequences

Consequences are a list of events that are likely to occur when patients follow or fail to follow their care plan. The most effective way to create this list is to review what could possibly be the outcome if the patient chooses to not follow their plan of care. With Beatrix, she enjoyed seeing Dr. Stein for her follow up appointments. She also knew she would disappoint him each time she reported she was not taking her medications. Listing the consequences of not following the care plan allows patients the opportunity to lay out what could happen from their perspective. We'll look at each of these as we complete the list and decide where the consequences are reinforcing or punishing.

Completing the list of consequences is done during a conversation with the patient and writing down their best guess of what might happen. Many of the consequences described in the "Don't Follow" list are avoided when listing the consequences in the "Follow" category.

When listing consequences, do not attempt to analyze them until everything that comes to mind is listed. The relative importance of each will become apparent as the PN/IF/LU/AN analysis is completed.

BEARS Targeted Consequence Analysis for Plan of Care

Patient Name	Beatriz		Target Behavior:		Take Prescobix 1 time daily
Date:	06/11/2016	Provider prescribing plan of care		Dr. Stein	
AdM Coach©	R. Wright, PhD, RN				

	ANTECEDENTS	BEHAVIOR	CONSEQUENCES	P	N	I	F	L	U	A	N
	Diagnosed with HIV Fear of death Family worried Fear of lost work Fear of disability May lose job	What may happen if I *don't follow* the Target Behavior described above?	Her doctor disappointed with her								
			HIV out of control								
			Disease gains power								
			Disease grow stronger								
			Medication loses potency								
			Run out of treatment options								
			No medication side effects								
			No cost for medications								
			Schedule not restricted by medications								
			Dr. may drop her from practice								
			Spouse nags' patient to take pills								
		BEHAVIOR	**CONSEQUENCES**	P	N	I	F	L	U	A	N
Plan of Care/HIV diagnosis	Visit to Drs. Office Diagnosis Prescription Teachback Counseling Disease symptoms Spouse nagging	What may happen if I *follow* the Target Behavior described above?	Stay out of trouble with doctor								
			HIV controlled better								
			No increase in disease power								
			Patient feels stronger								
			Medication keeps potency								
			Have treatment options								
			Has better health								
			High cost of medications								
			Take pills for lifetime								
			Provider experience								
			Spouse stops nagging								
			Dr. will keep treating her in practice								
			Have medication side effects								
		BEHAVIOR	**CONSEQUENCES**	P	N	I	F	L	U	A	N
	Fear of the unknown Beliefs	Disclose illness and seek counseling	New counselor will know information								
			May lose mother								
			May lose sister								
			May lose friends								
			Will cause shame								
			Fatalism (This is meant to be)								
			Husband engaged with family								

Consequences →	Strongest to Weakest Consequences								Extinction Consequences							
	PILA	NILA	PIUA	NIUA	PFLA	NFLA	PFUA	NFUA	PILN	NILN	PIUN	NIUN	PFLN	NFLN	PFUN	NFUN
	Most Power		Upper Middle		Lower Middle		Least Power		Least Weakness		Upper Middle		Lower Middle		Most Weakness	
Behavior(s)																
Non-Adherent																
Adherent																
Disclose Illness																

Determine Positive or Negative?

As a matter of convention, an AdM Coach will normally evaluate the four sets of possible consequence characteristics one category at a time. We will go through the listed consequences and first determine with the patient whether that particular consequence is positive or negative from the patient's perspective. So in the case of Dr. Stein's patient, first I would have a short conversation with "Beatriz" about the various definitions of POSITIVE and NEGATIVE. We would look at the synonyms. I would look at POSITIVE consequences as something that Beatriz has and/or wants and is willing to do a behavior to get or keep it. NEGATIVE consequences generally result in losing something that you have and/or receive something you don't want. For example, Beatriz's relationship with Dr. Stein is something she has and wants to continue. The consequence, "that Dr. Stein will be disappointed with her" is NEGATIVE. His approval will be taken away. The strength of the influence it has on her decision is yet to be determined.

Factors supporting non-adherence include three of the other primary consequences. These consequences contribute to the behavior of "she does not take her medication": it saves her money by not buying it, it reduces the possibilities for side-effects by not taking it, and it doesn't inconvenience her schedule or having to carry medications when it's time to take her pill. Three of the 11 (27%) consequences listed below on the BACA for non-adherence are analyzed as POSITIVE and support not following her care plan. On the other hand, 10 of the 13 listed consequences (77%) related to taking her medication (following the plan of care) are analyzed as POSITIVE and tend to support adherence. On an initial review of just POSITIVE and NEGATIVE, there appears to be a significant advantage for adherence. However, we have only looked at one of the four categories. As we work through the details, a clearer picture emerges.

BEARS Targeted Consequence Analysis for Plan of Care

Patient Name	Beatriz		Target Behavior:	Take Prescobix 1 time daily
Date:	06/11/2016	Provider prescribing plan of care	Dr. Stein	
AdM Coach©	R. Wright, PhD, RN			

ANTECEDENTS	BEHAVIOR	CONSEQUENCES	P	N	I	F	L	U	A	N
		Her doctor disappointed with her		X						
Diagnosed with HIV		HIV out of control		X						
Fear of death		Disease gains power		X						
Family worried	What may	Disease grow stronger		X						
Fear of lost work	happen if I *don't*	Medication loses potency		X						
Fear of disability	*follow* the Target	Run out of treatment options		X						
May lose job	Behavior	No medication side effects	X							
	described above?	No cost for medications	X							
		Schedule not restricted by medications	X							
		Dr. may drop her from practice		X						
		Spouse nags' patient to take pills		X						

ANTECEDENTS	BEHAVIOR	CONSEQUENCES	P	N	I	F	L	U	A	N
		Stay out of trouble with doctor	X							
Visit to Drs. Office		HIV controlled better	X							
Diagnosis		No increase in disease power	X							
Prescription		Patient feels stronger	X							
Teachback	What may	Medication keeps potency	X							
Counseling	happen if I *follow*	Have treatment options	X							
Disease symptoms	the Target	Has better health	X							
Spouse nagging	Behavior	High cost of medications		X						
	described above?	Take pills for lifetime		X						
		Provider experience	X							
		Spouse stops nagging	X							
		Dr. will keep treating her in practice	X							
		Have medication side effects		X						

ANTECEDENTS	BEHAVIOR	CONSEQUENCES	P	N	I	F	L	U	A	N
		New counselor will know information		X						
Fear of the		May lose mother		X						
unknown		May lose sister		X						
Beliefs	Disclose illness	May lose friends		X						
	and seek	Will cause shame		X						
	counseling	Fatalism (This is meant to be)		X						
		Husband engaged with family	X							

		Strongest to Weakest Consequences								Extinction Consequences						
Consequence →	PILA	NILA	PIUA	NIUA	PFLA	NFLA	PFUA	NFUA	PILN	NILN	PIUN	NIUN	PFLN	NFLN	PFUN	NFUN
	Most Power		Upper Middle		Lower Middle		Least Power		Least Weakness		Upper Middle		Lower Middle		Most Weakness	
Behavior(s)																
Non-Adherent																
Adherent																
Disclose Illness																

Determining Immediate or Future?

Timing of consequences is critical. Any consequence occurring during or immediately following a target behavior is significantly more powerful than a similar consequence occurring minutes, hours, days, or longer after the behavior. A patient who fails to take their medications today, may not see the consequence for that choice for up to three months until their next doctor visit. If Beatriz is non-adherent today, the consequence of having to face Dr. Stein's disappointment is in the future. Positive and Negative consequences lose their power when they are moved into the future. Positive/Immediate and Negative/Immediate are much more powerful in changing behavior than the promise of something good or the threat of something bad sometime in the future.

After completing the POSITIVE/NEGATIVE analysis, we then determine the timing of each consequence. As you can see in the BACA below, by filling in the next column of timing to determine whether each consequence is IMMEDIATE or FUTURE, another feature begins to emerge in the "don't follow" consequences. The three positive consequences are immediate while the potential threats from the disease are negative but in the future. Positive/Immediate consequences are more powerful than Negative/Future consequences.

The positive and negative nature of consequences are amended when time is considered. Positive/Immediate have a greater impact than Positive/Future consequences. For example, Beatriz's non-adherence (not taking her medication) has a significant impact on her finances from her perspective, because not having to spend money is Positive/Immediate.

Positive and negative outcomes are always important in predicting patient behavior. Timing adjusts the strength of these consequence. If a consequence is Negative or Positive and Future, it does not carry the same impact as a consequence that is Negative or Positive and will happen immediately after or as the patient is doing that behavior. Some of the patient's perspectives may not make sense from our perspective. In the "Follow" category Beatriz reported that her spouse stops nagging her when she takes her medications. She is avoiding something (nagging) that she doesn't want and it is immediate. This makes the consequence a POSITIVE/IMMEDIATE from her perspective.

As the RN AdM Coach analyzes the POSITIVE/FUTURE consequences, they will need to look for ways to add reinforcers that are more immediate to bolster the strength of these future consequences. Most medication regimens have future benefits, but future benefits do not necessarily support current behaviors. For example, Beatriz health improves and HIV related consequences are avoided when she takes her medications. These are positive outcomes, but they may not be appreciated for months or even years to come. In these instances, additional reinforcers must be added that have POSITIVE/IMMEDIATE consequences for her to stay on track in taking her medications.

Sharing information about her diagnosis with her family was out of the question from her perspective because in her mind they would reject her. The idea of using them as a support group, again from her perspective, is negative and immediate. It is unlikely she would avail herself of this important support group unless a more POSITIVE/IMMEDIATE reinforcer were added.

BEARS Targeted Consequence Analysis for Plan of Care

Patient Name	Beatriz		Target Behavior:	Take Prescobix 1 time daily
Date:	06/11/2016	Provider prescribing plan of care	Dr. Stein	
AdM Coach©	R. Wright, PhD, RN			

Plan of Care/HIV diagnosis

ANTECEDENTS	BEHAVIOR	CONSEQUENCES	P	N	I	F	L	U	A	N
Diagnosed with HIV Fear of death Family worried Fear of lost work Fear of disability May lose job	What may happen if I *don't follow* the Target Behavior described above?	Her doctor disappointed with her		X		X				
		HIV out of control		X		X				
		Disease gains power		X		X				
		Disease grow stronger		X		X				
		Medication loses potency		X		X				
		Run out of treatment options		X		X				
		No medication side effects	X		X					
		No cost for medications	X		X					
		Schedule not restricted by medications	X		X					
		Dr. may drop her from practice		X		X				
		Spouse nags' patient to take pills		X	X					

ANTECEDENTS	BEHAVIOR	CONSEQUENCES	P	N	I	F	L	U	A	N
Visit to Drs. Office Diagnosis Prescription Teachback Counseling Disease symptoms Spouse nagging	What may happen if I *follow* the Target Behavior described above?	Stay out of trouble with doctor	X			X				
		HIV controlled better	X			X				
		No increase in disease power	X			X				
		Patient feels stronger	X			X				
		Medication keeps potency	X			X				
		Have treatment options	X			X				
		Has better health	X			X				
		High cost of medications		X	X					
		Take pills for lifetime		X		X				
		Provider experience	X			X				
		Spouse stops nagging	X		X					
		Dr. will keep treating her in practice	X		X					
		Have medication side effects		X		X				

ANTECEDENTS	BEHAVIOR	CONSEQUENCES	P	N	I	F	L	U	A	N
Fear of the unknown Beliefs	Disclose illness and seek counseling	New counselor will know information		X	X					
		May lose mother		X	X					
		May lose sister		X	X					
		May lose friends		X	X					
		Will cause shame		X	X					
		Fatalism (This is meant to be)		X	X					
		Husband engaged with family	X		X					

Consequences →	Strongest to Weakest Consequences								Extinction Consequences							
	PILA	NILA	PIUA	NIUA	PFLA	NFLA	PFUA	NFUA	PILN	NILN	PIUN	NIUN	PFLN	NFLN	PFUN	NFUN
	Most Power		Upper Middle		Lower Middle		Least Power		Least Weakness		Upper Middle		Lower Middle		Most Weakness	
Behavior(s)																
Non-Adherent																
Adherent																
Disclose Illness																

Determine Whether the Consequence is Likely or Unlikely To Occur?

All consequences have a degree of probability as to whether each will occur or not. The greater the likelihood or "certainty", the more strength it has to influence the patient to do the behavior. LIKELY has replaced "Certain", as described by Dr. Daniels, because in medical practice, there are very few "certainties." The old saying regarding death and taxes reflect the only certain consequences of living. Medical recommendations in a plan of care, at least in the 21st Century, have a high likelihood of being successful. Consequences that are likely to occur have greater value in evaluating consequences than those that are unknown.

This third category of the BACA takes us closer to understanding how patients see the fallouts of "Following" or "Not Following" their care plan. Beatriz pointed out that disappointing Dr. Stein was Negative. At the same time, it was a Future event. It did not happen every time she skipped a dose of her medication. While he may be disappointed with her behavior. His disappointment will not be felt for days or weeks to come. In addition, he may not show any disappointment at all. He may simply pass it off as "Beatriz being Beatriz" and not make a big deal of it. In short, his disappointment is unknown – it may happen or it may not. This inability to predict a consequence is referred to as UNLIKELY. The NEGATIVE/FUTURE/UNLIKELY nature of this consequence is not very strong and will have little influence on her adherence.

Consequences that are LIKELY to happen have more power than an UNLIKELY consequence. Again it has to be paired with the other characteristics to understand the patient's priorities. Any consequence that is POSITIVE / IMMEDIATE / LIKELY to occur will get greater attention and have more influence than any future or unlikely consequence.

BEARS Targeted Consequence Analysis for Plan of Care

Patient Name	Beatriz	Target Behavior:	Take Prescobix 1 time daily
Date:	06/11/2016	Provider prescribing plan of care	Dr. Stein
AdM Coach©	R. Wright, PhD, RN		

Plan of Care/HIV diagnosis	ANTECEDENTS	BEHAVIOR	CONSEQUENCES	P	N	I	F	L	U	A	N
	Diagnosed with HIV Fear of death Family worried Fear of lost work Fear of disability May lose job	What may happen if I *don't follow* the Target Behavior described above?	Her doctor disappointed with her		X		X		X	X	
			HIV out of control		X		X	X			X
			Disease gains power		X		X	X			X
			Disease grow stronger		X		X	X			X
			Medication loses potency		X		X	X			X
			Run out of treatment options		X		X	X		X	
			No medication side effects	X		X		X		X	
			No cost for medications	X		X		X		X	
			Schedule not restricted by medications	X		X		X		X	
			Dr. may drop her from practice		X		X		X	X	
			Spouse nags' patient to take pills		X	X		X		X	
		BEHAVIOR	CONSEQUENCES	P	N	I	F	L	U	A	N
	Visit to Drs. Office Diagnosis Prescription Teachback Counseling Disease symptoms Spouse nagging	What may happen if I *follow* the Target Behavior described above?	Stay out of trouble with doctor	X			X		X	X	
			HIV controlled better	X			X		X		X
			No increase in disease power	X			X		X		X
			Patient feels stronger	X			X		X	X	
			Medication keeps potency	X			X		X		X
			Have treatment options	X			X		X	X	
			Has better health	X			X		X	X	
			High cost of medications		X	X			X	X	
			Take pills for lifetime		X		X	X		X	
			Provider experience		X		X	X		X	
			Spouse stops nagging		X	X		X		X	
			Dr. will keep treating her in practice	X		X		X		X	
			Have medication side effects		X		X	X		X	
		BEHAVIOR	CONSEQUENCES	P	N	I	F	L	U	A	N
	Fear of the unknown Beliefs	Disclose illness and seek counseling	New counselor will know information		X	X		X		X	
			May lose mother		X	X		X		X	
			May lose sister		X	X		X		X	
			May lose friends		X	X		X		X	
			Will cause shame		X	X		X		X	
			Fatalism (This is meant to be)		X	X		X		X	
			Husband engaged with family	X		X		X		X	

	Strongest to Weakest Consequences								Extinction Consequences							
Consequences	PILA	NILA	PIUA	NIUA	PFLA	NFLA	PFUA	NFUA	PILN	NILN	PIUN	NIUN	PFLN	NFLN	PFUN	NFUN
	Most Power		Upper Middle		Lower Middle		Least Power		Least Weakness		Upper Middle		Lower Middle		Most Weakness	
Behavior(s)																
Non-Adherent																
Adherent																
Disclose Illness																

Perception: Aware or Not Aware?

The fourth and final category pairing describes whether patients are *aware or not aware* of the consequence. This is a very unique and important component of medicine. The addition of AWARE/NOT AWARE to the BACA was necessary because many chronic and acute illnesses do not present signs or symptoms of the disease. Many medications and treatment options also do not exhibit any outward signs that they are working, from the patient's perspective. This leads patients to either not seek treatment for an illness they don't know they have or discontinue treatment believing it is ineffective. In applied behavior, doing an action, but not receiving any feedback for doing it, whether positive or negative, leads to an event called *"Extinction."* Behavior stops for lack of feedback.

Beatriz knows that not following her care plan is not good for treating her disease. The negative consequences are likely to occur, but are in the future. While she is AWARE of her disease, she is NOT AWARE that her viral load is increasing nor that her virus is becoming resistant to medications because of inconsistent compliance. She is not aware the disease is gaining power. In short, the disease process will progress outside of her level of perception, which will contribute to behavioral non-adherence and ultimately physical "Extinction."

Awareness also plays a massive role in medication adherence. Medication regimens to treat chronic diseases such as high blood pressure, diabetes, heart disease, HIV, etc. usually have long-term future outcomes, but the patient is unaware that the meds are working until lab tests are completed months into the future. These future outcomes, with no knowledge of their efficacy right now, lack the power that a rescue inhaler has on an asthmatic who is aware of the immediate relief or a patient with anaphylaxis who is aware of the immediate support by using their EpiPen.

This lack of awareness is a major contributor to why patients choose non-adherence. While the other categories are important factors to consider, the strength or weakness of a consequence can be directly affected by the patient's perception of its presence. When they take their medication, nothing happens. When they stop taking their medications, nothing happens. This lack of internal positive reinforcement leads to the extinction of the behavior of taking medications.

With Beatriz, we can see in the BACA that if she follows her treatment plan, her HIV is better controlled. That consequence is positive and yet the best outcome is a longer life (future). There tends to be no immediate consequence she can appreciate. It is unlikely, at this stage, to cure her disease and she is not aware the antiviral medications are quietly working. Anytime consequences are "covert" (that is, they are hidden from the patient's perception whether Positive or Negative), external positive reinforcement for doing the right behaviors must be built into the Adherence Improvement Plan. Anything less than external positive reinforcement, is inviting non-adherence to sit at the head of the table.

BEARS Targeted Consequence Analysis for Plan of Care

Patient Name	Beatriz		Target Behavior:	Take Prescobix 1 time daily
Date:	06/11/2016	Provider prescribing plan of care	Dr. Stein	
AdM Coach©	R. Wright, PhD, RN			

ANTECEDENTS	BEHAVIOR	CONSEQUENCES	P	N	I	F	L	U	A	N
Diagnosed with HIV, Fear of death, Family worried, Fear of lost work, Fear of disability, May lose job	What may happen if I *don't follow* the Target Behavior described above?	Her doctor disappointed with her		X		X		X	X	
		HIV out of control		X		X	X			X
		Disease gains power		X		X	X			X
		Disease grow stronger		X		X	X			X
		Medication loses potency		X		X	X			X
		Run out of treatment options		X		X	X		X	
		No medication side effects	X		X		X		X	
		No cost for medications	X		X		X		X	
		Schedule not restricted by medications	X		X		X		X	
		Dr. may drop her from practice		X		X		X	X	
		Spouse nags' patient to take pills		X	X		X		X	

ANTECEDENTS	BEHAVIOR	CONSEQUENCES	P	N	I	F	L	U	A	N
Visit to Drs. Office, Diagnosis, Prescription, Teachback, Counseling, Disease symptoms, Spouse nagging	What may happen if I *follow* the Target Behavior described above?	Stay out of trouble with doctor	X			X		X	X	
		HIV controlled better	X			X		X		X
		No increase in disease power	X			X		X		X
		Patient feels stronger	X			X		X	X	
		Medication keeps potency	X			X		X		X
		Have treatment options	X			X		X	X	
		Has better health	X			X		X	X	
		High cost of medications		X	X			X	X	
		Take pills for lifetime		X		X	X		X	
		Provider experience		X		X	X		X	
		Spouse stops nagging		X	X		X		X	
		Dr. will keep treating her in practice	X		X		X		X	
		Have medication side effects		X		X	X		X	

ANTECEDENTS	BEHAVIOR	CONSEQUENCES	P	N	I	F	L	U	A	N
Fear of the unknown, Beliefs	Disclose illness and seek counseling	New counselor will know information		X	X		X		X	
		May lose mother		X	X		X		X	
		May lose sister		X	X		X		X	
		May lose friends		X	X		X		X	
		Will cause shame		X	X		X		X	
		Fatalism (This is meant to be)		X	X		X		X	
		Husband engaged with family	X		X		X		X	

(Left vertical label: Plan of Care/HIV diagnosis)

	Strongest to Weakest Consequences								Extinction Consequences							
Consequences →	PILA	NILA	PIUA	NIUA	PFLA	NFLA	PFUA	NFUA	PILN	NILN	PIUN	NIUN	PFLN	NFLN	PFUN	NFUN
	Most Power		Upper Middle		Lower Middle		Least Power		Least Weakness		Upper Middle		Lower Middle		Most Weakness	
Behavior(s)																
Non-Adherent																
Adherent																
Disclose Illness																

Seeing The Whole Picture.

After completing the BACA analysis, shorthand abbreviations are used to get a comprehensive picture of how each consequence affects the patient's ability to follow their care plan. PN/IF/LU/AN are the initials for each category pair and are used to abbreviate each consequence.

At the bottom of the BACA, the number of each consequence is tallied and the strength of all the consequences are evaluated. For example, the consequences that have the most powerful effect on adherence are PILAs and NILAs, which stand for POSITIVE/IMMEDIATE/LIKELY/AWARE and NEGATIVE/IMMEDIATE/LIKELY/AWARE. These two consequences will either greatly strengthen a behavior to happen again or greatly hinder it from happening again. The different consequences vary in influence. Consequences that end in A (AWARE), vary the influence of the consequence on getting the behavior to increase or decrease. Consequences that end in N (NOT AWARE), determine how much influence that consequence has on putting that behavior on extinction. In other words, the behavior just fades away.

What Does It All Mean?

Learning what rewards or punishes patients as they look at their prescriptions or treatment plans is something that has not been consciously done throughout history. Healthcare providers assume everyone wants to get better, and they do. The question is this. Are they willing to pay the price or more accurately, do the behavioral things necessary to achieve a future better outcome? The BEARS Adherence Consequence Analysis (BACA) provides the necessary baseline for deciding how to create new habits that replace a lifetime of reliable, but harmful, old habits.

Taking pills for a lifetime may be considered a negative event that is immediately "punishing" from the patient's perspective and yet, result in positive outcomes in the future. The trick is to know that in advance.

Non-adherence is a "today" event. *Behavior goes where reinforcement flows and all behavior returns to baseline without positive reinforcement.* Few care plans offer positive reinforcement. Symptoms may be hidden. The effects of treatment may be hidden. The behavioral baseline for most people does not include taking medications. Believing that patient education will change behavior and repeated exposure to medical brochures will create new habits, shows a basic lack of understanding on why people do the things they do.

Adherence Management Coaching (AdM Coach) provides clinicians and family members with a toolkit that avoids what Mark Twain said, "…tossing [patients] out the window but coaxes (reinforces) them (their adherence) downstairs one step at a time." It also avoids the Cheshire Cat's warning about the paths they intend to take. If you know where you are going (following their care plan) then the adherence path will get you there. Finally, as Twain remarked, "I can go for two months on a good compliment!" The Adherence Improvement Plan (AIP) ensures that patient compliments are closer and more frequent than two-months apart.

The key to success is found in ensuring desired behaviors are reinforced at every opportunity. Look for any undesired behaviors that are being reinforced. Look for cues in the home environment that encourage old habits? These have to be identified and removed. If a patient had a habit of having coffee in the morning with a cigarette on the porch, consider moving the morning coffee to another location.

People don't change or develop new habits because, "they want it badly enough." Desire plays a very minor role. Habits are changed because they are reinforced. The actions to get a new habit started may take a lot of reinforcing. Over time the reinforcing schedule can be thinned, but not removed. If reinforcers are removed completely, you can expect the void to be filled with the return of old bad habits.

The following Table provides the map in addressing consequences for patient adherence.

To increase adherent behaviors...

1. Provide more PILA* Consequences and PIUA** consequences for adherent behavior.
2. Provide more Antecedents (Cues for desired behavior.
3. Link Antecedents for adherent behaviors with positive consequences.
4. Eliminate as many Negative (punishing) consequences for adherent behaviors as possible (e.g., inconvenience, expenses, side effects).

To decrease non-adherent behaviors...

5. Eliminate as many Positive (reinforcing) consequences for non-adherent behavior as you can.
6. Eliminate as many Antecedents for non-adherent behaviors as possible.

*PILA - Positive, Immediate, Likely, Aware
**PIUA Positive, Immediate, Unlikely, Aware

Key points:

- RN AdM Coaches© will accomplish the following:

- Identify at-risk patients (B-MAAS),

- Determine physical and intellectual impairments that may contribute to non-adherence (B-PAAS),

- Evaluate care plans with patients to find consequences that punish patients (BACA),

- Work with clinicians to make appropriate changes where possible to reduce "punishing" consequences,

- Work with patients, families and clinicians to develop and implement an Adherence Improvement Plan (AIP),

- Look for hidden symptoms and hidden results and share those with clinicians to see where possible changes can be made or reinforcers added.

Persistence vs. Extinction:
The Long Haul Of Adherence

Adherence is "sticking to the plan," while "persistence" suggests that the plan will last more than a few days or weeks. In many instances, persistence might be the remainder of the patient's life. As can be seen in the following graphic, many patients become significantly non-adherent, starting the day after discharge. This slide represents a high cost in terms of potential unnecessary readmissions and acute care episodes.

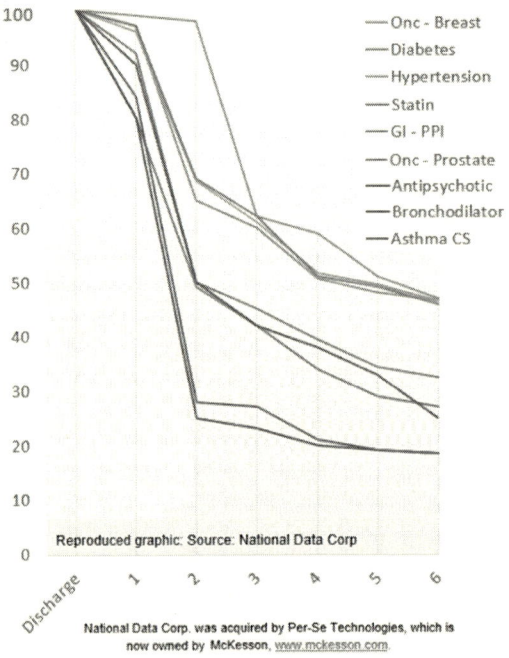

The long-term cause of non-persistence can likely be placed in the reality that nothing is going on to reinforce patient adherent behavior. Regardless of the diagnosis and treatment, each medical issue shows a significant drop off in adherence at the two-month mark. The trend line, although stopped by this author after six months, continues to decline in each area over the next eight months.

The conclusion of causality can only point to the lack of reinforcement in every category. Many patients reported they abandoned their treatment plan because they did not feel any better. If side effects accompanied the medications, cost, or inconvenience, staying on their medication was more punishing than reinforcing. Following a fundamental law of behavior, "behavior goes where reinforcement flows," it's no wonder that adherence dropped off considerably after two months.

There is a common misconception concerning consequences. Consequences tend to be thought of as always punishing. For example, the person does something he is not supposed to, and thus, he gets something that he doesn't want. Consequences that are punishing are often much less effective than other consequences. The consequences that are more useful and effective are those that are positively reinforcing (rewarding).

Before we begin to look at a typical consequence, we can first look at consequences in our everyday lives.

Typical Consequence Example 1: Let's look back at the previous speeding example. You're speeding down the highway and see a police car. You don't hit the brakes but instead keep speeding. The police officer puts on a siren, pulls you over and gives you a ticket. What are the behavior and the consequences? The behavior was you continued to speed, and the result was you getting a ticket. The next time you're speeding and see a police officer, are you going to keep speeding? Probably not. You are less likely to speed in front of the police officer because you received a ticket. Therefore, the consequence (getting a ticket) of this behavior (speeding) may cause you to not engage in the same behavior (speeding in front of a police officer) in the future.

Typical Consequence Example 2: Let's look back at the umbrella example. It is raining outside, so you get your umbrella and open it. You walk in the rain, and you don't get wet. What is the behavior and the consequence? The behavior is opening the umbrella and the result is that you don't get wet. Next time it is raining outside you are more likely to use an umbrella so that you don't get wet. Therefore, the consequence (not getting wet) of this behavior (opening your umbrella) may cause you to engage in the same behavior (using an umbrella) in the future.

Typical Consequence Examples 3: You forget to pay your credit card bill. On your statement, there is a $100 late charge. What is the behavior, and what is the consequence? The behavior is forgetting to pay your credit card bill, and the result is the $100 late charge. Next time you get your credit card statement, are you likely to pay your bill? You're more likely to pay your bill on time. Therefore, the consequence (the $100 late fee) of this behavior (forgetting to pay your bill) may cause you to pay your bill on time in the future. Now let's look at some typical consequences with family members.

Family Member Example 1: You take your prescription to the pharmacy to get it filled. The pharmacist tells you the medication will cost $175.00. The patient knows this is a medication that he/she will be on for the rest of his/her life. This person is on a fixed income. The consequence ($175) of filling this prescription (behavior) is that he/she may not be able to pay the rent or have to sacrifice in some other area. The results of not taking the medication may be years away. The results of not paying the rent are immediate eviction. What are the behavior and the consequence? The behavior is getting the prescription filled, and the consequence is sticker shock. Is this person more or less likely to fill prescriptions in the future?

Family Member Example 2: The patient gets the materials together to give himself an insulin injection. He finishes the injection, and you say, "great job! You did each step perfectly." What is the behavior and the consequence? The behavior is giving the injection, and the consequence is the praise "great job! You did each step perfectly." Is this patient more or less likely to correctly give himself insulin on his own in the future?

Family Member Example 3: A patient cleans her wound. To reward her, you immediately join her for a cup of coffee. This is one of her favorite activities. What is the behavior, and what is the consequence? The action is cleaning the wound, and the result is getting to have coffee with someone. Is this patient more or less likely to properly clean her injury in the future as a result of being rewarded? The consequence (having coffee) of the behavior (cleaning her wounds) may cause the patient to clean her wound again in the future properly.

Sometimes the consequences that follow a behavior are arranged. That is, we set up a situation in which we can control the consequences. Sometimes the consequences that follow behavior are natural. For example, if you touch a hot stove, the consequence will be that you will immediately get burned. Sometimes the consequences that follow a behavior are socially mediated. That is, the result is delivered by someone else as in the case of wound care and, "great job!"

Key points:

- Consequences are things in the environment that happen right after behavior.

- Consequences are to be described factually.

- Consequences can be natural, socially mediated, or arranged.

- Consequences control or influence behavior.

- Consequences are not always punishing. The most effective consequences are those that are rewarding.

Now It's Your Turn:

- List a consequence that you can control.

- List a consequence that is a positive reinforcer.

- List a consequence that is naturally occurring.

Can't Or Won't Behaviors

When you've seen one patient response to a request, you've only seen one response. Depending on where you live, the US is rapidly becoming a very diverse country.

Added to this diversity is the reality of all the illnesses that plague us. In the "Velluvial Matrix," as described by Dr. Atul Gawande, there are 13,600 ways our bodies can fail us, 6,000 medications, and over 4,000 procedures to medicate and treat them. No other business is more complex nor can do greater good… or harm than healthcare.

What is the Function of this Patient's Non-Adherence?

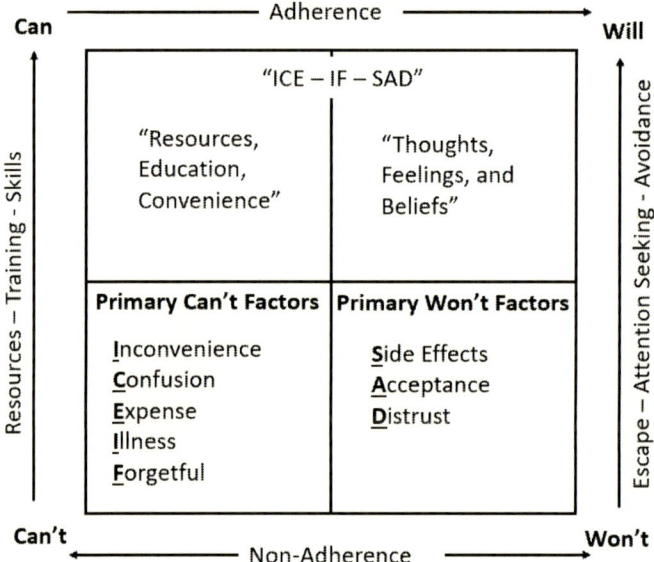

The formula for misunderstanding each other has grown exponentially. Regardless of each of the almost 200 cultural variables spread across this land, patients will initially fall into one of four categories when it comes to following their plan of care. Some of your patients CAN and WILL initially follow their plan of care. Another group CAN, but WON'T follow their care plan. Another population CAN'T, for some resource issue but WILL if the resource issues were addressed. The last group is CAN'T and WON'T, period!

In the absence of organic brain disease, "forgetful" patients are using the term as a "bridge excuse" for not wanting to deal with one or more of the significant three issues: inconvenience, expense and side effects.

"Forgetfulness" should be a red flag to dig a little deeper. If these issues can be resolved, there is an opportunity to move them to the CAN and WILL population.

Illness presents as another challenge in the shortlist of excuses as to why patients choose to be non-adherent. This population is made of patients who have no symptoms and don't believe there is something dangerous, slowly damaging their health. They may have the resources necessary to be adherent; they don't have sufficient evidence they are ill, and, as is often the case, their managing medications work quietly and without fanfare. This reinforces their belief that they are okay.

The other side of the adherence coin is persistence. The behavioral Law of Extinction offers some understanding of why patients stop taking medications.

Human Repertoire.

Every behavior in the human repertoire has consequences. These consequences can either increase behavior (e.g., positive and negative reinforcement), or they can decrease and stop the behavior (punishers and penalties). In the following sections, we'll take a closer look at each of these areas to ensure that AdM Home Coaches have a clear understanding of the different consequences and how they can be used to either strengthen or weaken behaviors.

As complex as disease, treatments, and the health services delivery system are, knowing how to change patient behavior effectively gives AdM Home Coaches a decided advantage over other forms of patient education.

The Ethics Of Behavior Change.

Over the years, some people have questioned the ethics of health services clinicians, making a deliberate attempt to change a patient's habits. The emergence of the Adherence Management Coaching© approach in the

21st Century places the focus of the science of applied behavior analysis on strengthening adherence to a patient's plan of care.

In the late 1960s and 70s, behavior modification emerged as the most effective way to teach skills to children on the autism spectrum. Over the years, the term was deemed to be too draconian, and behavior analysis emerged and has remained the acceptable term through the 1980's where Drs. Aubrey Daniels and Jon Bailey expanded the science into the workplace.

The term behavior analysis was frowned upon for similar reasons. Employers viewed science as too invasive. Their focus, according to Dr. Daniels, was improved performance, and thus, in the early 1990's "Performance Management" was coined and over the past almost forty years, this industry has embraced the scientific approach to worker safety and improved productivity.

Patient education programs have embraced Teachback as the primary means of introducing clinical information and care plan understanding to patients. For thirty-five years, tens of thousands of nurses and clinicians have used Teachback with millions of patients. The goal with Teachback was that patients could voice back their understanding of their discharge plan. Motivational Interviewing (MI) is another tool in the patient adherence bag that focuses on changing beliefs and attitudes about items in the discharge plan that patients were ambivalent about. MI trained clinicians focused on helping patients explore and resolve their ambivalence in a non-confrontational manner.

Medication Therapy Management (MTM) , "…encourages patients to take an active role in managing their medications." From the time that medicine became patient-focused, and perhaps before then, there has been a concerted effort to change patient's habits. Until the emergence of AdM Home Coaching, programs have focused on processes, feelings, beliefs, and antecedents (e.g., bottles, blister packs, and buzzers). AdM Home Coaches learn how to focus on adherence and to reinforce the tasks necessary to move the bar in favor of health-improving habits.

Reinforcement

The only way to change desired behavior is to use positive reinforcement. Reinforcement is the subject of this chapter. As previously stated, reinforcers are consequences that follow behavior, and because of the reinforcer, behavior is more likely to occur again in the future. While reinforcers are typically pleasant or desirable, this is not always the case. Therefore, it is essential to remember that for consequences to be reinforcing, the pinpoint behavior must be more likely to occur in the future. Think of reinforcers as what we use to motivate patients to engage in adherent behavior.

Often, the reinforcer is an addition to the environment or something that patients receive (R+) as a result of engaging in adherent behavior. In Appendix E is a list of possible reinforcers that may be given to patients and categories they may fall under. It is called the BEARS Reinforcement Survey.

Sometimes the reinforcer is something that is removed, avoided, or taken away (R-), and thus patients are more likely to engage in that same behavior in the future. With these reinforcers, patients are rewarded by getting out of doing things (task, duties, chores, etc.) or gets away from people he or she does not like or people that are associated with punishment. Typically, the item to be removed is something or someone that the patient has an aversion to or does not like.

Reinforcers differ from person-to-person. In other words, what will increase behavior for one patient will not necessarily increase behavior with another.

Be aware that just as reinforcers differ from one person to another, not all items, objects, or activities that are reinforcing right now, will be reinforcing in 10 minutes. Using a small number of reinforcers can decrease the likelihood that patients will lose motivation or preference for the item.

A patient's preferences change from moment to moment, and we need to be aware of this fact. For example, a person whose reinforcer is chocolate chip cookies may not be interested in them or may not want them immediately after lunch. In this case, you'll have to find something else to use as a reinforcer. The challenge for AdM Coaches is to find the most effective reinforcer at that moment in time. Remember that items and activities are only a reinforcer if they increase behavior. The methods for identifying reinforcers are listed below. Please refer to Appendix E for a Reinforcer Survey example.

Key points:

- We all behave to get something or to get out of something.

- Be able to identify things patients can get by engaging in a behavior.

- Be able to identify things that patients can get out of by engaging in a behavior.

- Reinforcers differ from person to person.

- Not all items are reinforcing all the time.

- Items and activities are only reinforcers if they increase behavior

Now It's Your Turn:

- Think of and write down three things that could be used to reinforce your behavior.

- Write down three things your patient would want as a reinforcer to stay healthy.

Reinforcing Adherence – Getting Patients From Prescription To Persistence.

There is no other patient care topic, with more written about it than what to do with people who choose not to follow their care plan. Civil trial courts enjoy the ability to describe "the reasonably prudent person." In their text, writers describe how a reasonably prudent person would behave, given a specific set of criteria, and in an accurately described environment. Any deviation, from what a reasonably prudent person would do, places the errant person at legal risk. The rule of law offers a standard that all people, regardless of gender, race, religious background, and cultural variables, can recognize and follow. When the errant behaver chooses not to follow the rules, if caught, they must deal with the consequences.

One might believe that people who are ill might be considered "reasonably prudent patients" if they follow their plan of care. They did, after all, have symptoms, saw a physician, received a diagnosis, and got a care plan. Why would anyone choose to ignore the medical advice they sought out? Why, given their diagnosis, would reasonably prudent people want not to do behaviors that could add months or years of healthy living to their lives?

I recently read an article in a prestigious journal that said, "If you want to improve adherence, look for patients who are adherent." Frankly, that advice is less than helpful. It is the defeatist who believes that nothing can be done to improve adherence. If you want to improve adherence, define the desired clinical outcomes, describe the behaviors necessary to achieve those results, and reinforce those behaviors. Behavior goes where reinforcement flows. Results follow behavior. Just keep in mind that in the absence of reinforcers and punishers to make us aware of our disease, extinction of adherent behaviors is possible.

Reinforce The Behavior - Outcomes Will Follow

Positive reinforcers (R+) that immediately follow a target behavior increase the likelihood of a behavior occurring again. Pill-taking is a behavior, while normal blood pressures, reduced viral loads, normal A1C levels, and normal lipid levels are all outcomes.

Adherence management defines the desired clinical outcomes and then describes the behaviors necessary to achieve those results. Pill-taking and exercise are behaviors. They can be reinforced every day. Results or outcomes may take weeks or months. Reinforce the behavior, and then celebrate the outcomes that follow.

For countless decades, various researchers, authors, clinicians, and a shaman or two have offered their surefire solution to improve adherence. From 1818 to 1918, we began to see the scientific application of education to the training of physicians and treatment facilities. From 1918 to 2000, particularly in the War years, revealed an exponential growth in medicines, procedures, quality assurance. Yet non-adherence, despite our best efforts in motivation and education, persisted at levels much the same as it was in the days of Hippocrates (460-370 BCE).

Between 2000 and 2018, there was a renewed effort at increasing motivation and education to combat non-adherence. Medication management and medication reconciliation have reduced harm to patients, and yet non-adherence is still an important topic of concern with increased patient morbidity and mortality, increased costs to hospitals with unplanned readmissions, increased costs to third-party payers, and lost revenues to big pharma. To quote Drs. Aubrey Daniels and Darnell Lattal, " The only way people will ever reach their potential is through the effective use of positive reinforcement."[2]

People are patients for short episodes throughout their lives. Clinical professionals believe people will automatically go along with clinical recommendations. About half the time they are right. That leaves a tremendous opportunity to change the other half of patient behaviors.

How Do We Determine What's Reinforcing?

Remember, reinforcers differ from patient to patient. Reinforcers are typically items, objects, or activities that patients like or enjoy. With some patients, you can ask them what they want or what they like, and they will tell you. However, remember that if your patient is a family member, they might be

2   A Daniels, D Lattal, Life's a PICNIC... When you understand behavior, Sloan Publishing Hudson, NY

vague or unclear about their wants and needs. When this is the case, we need to figure out what their reinforcers are in other ways.

One way we can do this is to ask relatives or other people who know the patient well, including fellow AdM Home Coaches, about the patient's likes, dislikes, and preferences. This is referred to as the interview method.

We can also watch what patients do. Look to see what items, objects, or activities a patient spends time doing, eating, or drinking. Typically, the thing or activity is something they like, and then you can use this as a reinforcer. This is the observation method.

Another method is to provide your patients with selections. You can show a patient two or more objects and let him or her pick one. The patient may tell you or name the object he or she prefers. This is the selection method.

Key points:

- Ask friends, relatives, fellow AdM Home Coaches, or other people who know your patient well about the patient's likes, dislikes, and preferences (interview method).
- Watch what the patient does (observation method).
- Provide selections (selection method).

Now It's Your Turn:

- List four reinforcers you obtained from interviewing.
- List four reinforcers you obtained from observing someone.
- List four reinforcers you obtained from providing selections.

Joy, Pleasure, Satisfaction – The Path To Meaningful Reinforcers.

Everyone knows what they like or what provides some joy, pleasure, or satisfaction. The question is, have they ever taken the time to write them down? For more than a year, I asked new employees during their onboarding process what they liked or to list things that were worth earning. Initially, each person would have a difficult time recording what they wanted. As the old saying goes, it was like pulling teeth. When you have seen one person's list of reinforcers, you have seen one person's list.

I have an identical twin brother, and our list of reinforcers is significantly different. While we might have some things in common, he might say that one item I found gave me pleasure, gave him satisfaction. Many people looking for reinforcers don't take the time to break down their reinforcers into joy, pleasure, or satisfaction subgroups. The value of reinforcers will change from time to time. Starting the reinforcement process by using the highest value reinforcer can lead to dissatisfaction. When the highest value reinforcer is used and the patient becomes satiated with it, then the next choice is of lower value, leading to less success, not higher.

We break reinforcers into three categories for this reason. There are days when a reinforcer that gives "joy" is of higher value than one that gives pleasure or satisfaction. On other days, doing something that results in satisfaction may be lower on the list of benefits but, at that time, it is more reinforcing than either joy or pleasure.

Social And Tangible Reinforcers – Choosing The Right One.

Most of us can remember as children the words, "Mom (or Dad) look at me!" As you excitedly did some behavior like jumping or diving in a pool. That glance from your parent was sufficient to reinforce that behavior. Social reinforcers from significant other people in our lives are often the mainstay of desired behavior. The key is that social reinforcers are readily available and usually either not delivered or delivered too late to be an effective reinforcer. Mark Twain is quoted to have said, "I can go for two months on a good compliment." Such is the power of positive social reinforcement.

Tangible reinforcers are things of modest value, such as food, money, trophies, t-shirts, etc. that can be earned to increase behavior and celebrate outcomes. Social and tangible reinforcers depend on the behavior of the patient as well as the behavior of someone else giving out the reinforcer (such as a physician, nurse educator, AdM Coach, or family member.) Social or tangible reinforcers are necessary when natural reinforcers do not produce the target behavior. All social and most tangible reinforcers are created reinforcers that are purposely crafted to shape certain target behaviors to improve adherence.

Natural reinforcers do not depend on the presence of another person. When our interactions with machines (such as appliances, tools, automobiles, computers, etc.) or with our environment provide us with feedback on what we expect and desire, they are called naturally reinforcing. No one needs to observe or measure our behavior to determine the effectiveness of the naturally reinforcing consequence for the behavior to continue or increase.

Air is naturally reinforcing. If you don't believe me, hold your breath. Your body will let you know when you need to increase your behavior of breathing again (or you will pass out and your body will take over for you anyway.) Turning the handle on a faucet (behavior) produces water (R+). The water coming out is a reinforcer for the behavior of turning the handle. Turning the handle produces water immediately and with a high degree of certainty. It is naturally reinforcing and is all that is needed to maintain or increase the behavior.

Sacrifice And Satiation – Increasing And Decreasing The Value Of Reinforcers.

For reinforcers to be "reinforcing," they must have value for each individual patient and the reinforcer is not readily available from another source other than the AdM Coach. If, for example, ice cream is always available to anyone who asks for it and your patient is unwilling to give up that availability unless it is earned, it cannot be used as a reinforcer. A patient must be willing to sacrifice a reinforcer should s/he not preform the required behavior associated with receiving that reinforcer. Primary reinforcers have nature-driven value. Food, water, air, sleep, and sex are natural reinforcers for all people. Food and liquids are the only two primary reinforcers that can be manipulated with any effectiveness (e.g., reservations at a favorite restaurant, a bottle of favorite beverage). Each must be withheld and earned for achieving adherence goals. Sex, when appropriately offered, is a most powerful reinforcer. Ensure it is reinforcing to both partners. When sex is reinforcing for one and punishing for the other partner, you will likely not get the desired results. Look for secondary reinforcers. Relief from pain, while not a primary reinforcer, is a common event that people commonly seek to reduce or avoid. Splinting, taking analgesics, and not touching hot objects are negatively reinforced learned behaviors that people do. These prevent or reduce pain.

The difference between positive and negative reinforcers is that negative reinforcement changes behavior to avoid an unwanted consequence. Positive reinforcement changes behavior because a person is getting something s/he wants or needs as a consequence of doing the desired behavior. Negative reinforcement is effective when the consequence is immediate. Wearing a jacket to avoid the cold is immediate. Rescue inhalers are reinforcing if airways are opened immediately. Blood pressure medications are designed to prevent hypertension and stroke and are "negatively reinforcing." The reason non-adherence is more likely, with hypertension and many long-term medications, is the consequences are likely months, years, or even decades in the future. Consequences that are positive but happen in the future require their behaviors to be reinforced more readily in the present (i.e. pill-taking for future benefit.)

Another concept of positive reinforcers is satiation. Satiation is when a patient has had too much of a reinforcer and the item is no longer reinforcing. Think about your last big meal (holidays are a good example.) Once you are completely stuffed with dinner and can't eat another bite, will bringing out another serving bowl of mashed potatoes be very reinforcing for you to do a desired behavior? Maybe, if the behavior is to leave the table to avoid the pain of stuffing more food in an already satiated stomach. When satiation occurs, the reinforcer is no longer valuable as a reinforcer until some time has passed without it and the value returns.

When Do I Give A Patient A Reinforcer?

There are two methods for when to give patients reinforcers. The first way is to provide a patient a reinforcer immediately following a specific target behavior. This method requires a behavior to occur first and then the reinforcer is given. This method is called contingent reinforcement. A reinforcer is delivered to the patients after all clinical skill acquisitions have been accomplished. This would be considered contingent reinforcement. Receiving the reinforcer is contingent upon doing the behavior.

When delivering reinforcement that requires a response or behavior, at first, you may give your patient the reinforcer at every response or behavior to ensure compliance or competency in the new skill or behavior. As the patient masters the new behavior you would give the patient a reinforcer occasionally. Giving a reinforcer at every response or behavior is called continuous reinforcement and is typically used to teach new or difficult tasks. Only giving a reinforcer sometimes or after a random number of responses or behaviors is called intermittent reinforcement and is used for skills that patient can already do or are easy.

The second method to give your patient reinforcers is not requiring any targeted behavior, response, or task. This method is called the non-contingent reinforcement. Non-contingent reinforcement is "something for nothing." That is, they don't have to earn it. The only requirement for delivering reinforcement non-contingently is that the patient is not engaging in any non-adherent or problem behavior. It's a positive reward for refraining from unwanted behavior over some period of time. Taking a child for ice cream at the end of the week for not fighting with their sister during that same week. It is used as a reinforcer for not doing an unwanted behavior.

Non-contingent reinforcement is essential for developing and maintaining an adherent relationship with the patient, while at the same time establishing the AdM Coach as the primary source of positive reinforcement.

The combination of delivering unearned reinforcers and earned reinforcers for specific behaviors, will teach the patient that he or she gets reinforcing things from you. This will ultimately make the patient more likely to follow your directions and less likely to engage in problem behaviors with you.

Regardless of when you reinforce a patient, always remember that each time you give a patient an item, object, or activity, you should always pair it with social praise. For example, if a patient self-medicates appropriately, then you'll want to say something like, "you are doing a great job with your medication schedule."

Other examples of social praise include:

> Way to go recording your blood pressure.
>
> Great job cleaning your ileostomy.
>
> Good following directions.
>
> Awesome exercise program today.

Key points:

- Contingent reinforcement requires a patient to do a behavior or give a response to do a specific task before the reinforcer is delivered.

- Be able to demonstrate delivering reinforcement contingent upon a behavior happening.

- Continuous reinforcement is when a reinforcer is given after every response or behavior.

- Continuous reinforcement is used when teaching new or difficult tasks. Use intermittent reinforcement after acquiring the new behavior.

- Be able to demonstrate delivering reinforcement continuously and/or intermittently.

Now It's Your Turn:
- List when you would deliver a contingent reinforcement.
- List when you would deliver a non-contingent reinforcement.

Effectiveness Of Reinforcement.

When we look at the effectiveness of reinforcement, we're looking at how likely the behavior is to occur again in the future. The more likely the behavior is to happen again, the more effective the reinforcer is.

Five things can influence how effective a reinforcer is.

Immediacy.

Remember that reinforcement is a carefully thought out procedure used to increase the occurrence of adherent behaviors. For reinforcers to be effective, reinforcers must be delivered immediately after the behavior you are trying to reinforce. For example, if the behavior that you are trying to increase is your patient taking medications as prescribed, you would reinforce a patient immediately after he or she takes their medication. If you wait or fail to reinforce the behavior, it will not be as effective in increasing behavior.

Although we should always try to get a reinforcer immediately after the behavior you are trying to increase; sometimes, the reinforcer cannot be delivered promptly. Provide praise for the behavior and then reinforce the behavior as quickly as possible. By always pairing the item with social approval, the social consent serves as a signal that the reinforcer is coming.

Size.

The size of the reinforcer can influence whether it will increase behavior. First, the size of the reinforcer should be limited. For edible reinforcers, this may mean a piece of the food item instead of the whole food item (i.e., a bit of cookie and not an entire cookie). For activity-based reinforcers, this may mean limiting the amount of time patients can participate in an activity (1 minute instead of 5 minutes). By providing smaller reinforcers, patients will avoid becoming satiated. Remember, satiation is when a patient has had too much of a reinforcer and that reinforcer has lost its value and is no longer reinforcing. For some people, it may take a long time before they have had too much of the same item, while for others it may only take a short amount of time. This is very patient specific and something you'll discover as you work with your patient.

Variety.

Another thing we can do to make sure reinforcers are effective is to provide a variety of reinforcers. If patients are interested and reinforced by several items at the same time, changing the reinforcers that are delivered can also increase the effectiveness of the reinforcers. If you use the same reinforcer all day long, by the end of the day, those items will no longer be reinforcing.

When this occurs, patients become satiated on that item. Occasionally, however, patient may not be interested in a variety of reinforcers at the same time. When this occurs, there are things you can try to vary the reinforcer.

Sometimes, there are natural opportunities to change the reinforcer. For example, if a reinforcer is a food item, you can almost guarantee that eventually, a patient will need a drink of some sort (especially if the food item is extremely salty). When this occurs, it provides a natural opportunity to vary the reinforcer from food to water.

Deprivation.

Reinforcers are most effective if a patient has not had them in some time; that is, if they have gone through a period without having a particular item, object, or activity. This principle is called deprivation and comes into play in the above food example. Since the patient has been eating the food item for a lengthy period, he or she has been deprived of a drink; therefore, the drink is more reinforcing at that moment and more effective at increasing behavior. Do not confuse the concept of deprivation with the action of deprivation. We do not deprive patients of items they need or choose. Instead, in certain instances, patients may not have selected an item for some period of time having deprived themselves of that item, and therefore, that item becomes more reinforcing than others. Patients must be willing to give up reinforcing items until they earn them.

Effort.

The last thing we can do to maximize the effectiveness of reinforcement is to examine how much effort patients put forth to get reinforcement. In other words, is a patient working very hard for too little reinforcement, or is the patient not working hard enough for too much reinforcement, etc. There's a delicate balance between the amount of effort required for patients to respond and the amount of reinforcement he or she should receive for that response.

Key points:

There are five areas you can change to maximize reinforcer effectiveness.

- Immediacy.
- Size.
- Variety.
- Deprivation.
- Effort.
- Deliver reinforcement immediately (generally within 2 seconds), and pair a reinforcer with social praise.
- All reinforcers must be of an appropriate size.
- Reinforcers should be varied to maintain or maximize their effectiveness.

- The effort of the task should be balanced with the amount of reinforcement. More effort, more reinforcement.

- Deprivation is when a patient has not had an item or object for some time; thus, it increases its value.

Now It's Your Turn:

- List two examples of delivering appropriate size reinforcement.

- List two examples of using a variety of reinforcers.

- List two examples of delivering reinforcement based on patient effort.

Differential Reinforcement.

Differential reinforcement is providing different levels of reinforcement for different behaviors. We explained earlier the difference between adherent (appropriate) behavior and non-adherent (inappropriate) behavior. Using differential reinforcement, we provide reinforcement of the adherent behavior and no reinforcement for non-adherent behavior. In this manner, we can increase adherent behavior and decrease the non-adherent behavior.

Differential reinforcement can also apply to how we reinforce an adherent patient's behavior. For example, if a patient is engaged in adherent behavior without prompting, we should provide reinforcement. However, if the patient is involved in a task with prompting, we would still reinforce, but would not give as much reinforcement as we would if the task had been done independently. You always want to strengthen independent behavior or behaviors that the patient does without our help more than any task or behavior that requires or prompting or support.

Do not confuse this concept of differential reinforcement with continuous reinforcement that we discussed earlier. Continuous reinforcement refers to how often we reinforce the behavior, and differential reinforcement refers to how much reinforcement we give for each behavior.

Key points:

- Differential reinforcement is the concept of providing different amounts, levels, or types of reinforcement for prompted vs. independent behaviors.

- Using differential reinforcement reinforces preferred behaviors and limits reinforcing inappropriate behaviors.

- Using differential reinforcement, reinforce independent responses more heavily than responses that require help or prompting.

Now It's Your Turn:

- List two examples of differential reinforcement that you use every day.

Documenting And Graphing Care Plans And Adherence Plans

Care Plans: Remember the ABCs of behavior? Think of medical discharge plans or care plans in terms of antecedents, behaviors, and consequences.

A care plan is an antecedent or cue or instructions that are given to a patient to perform certain behaviors that all have certain consequences. The guidance tells patients what behaviors he/she is to perform at a specific point in time. While we use cues all the time, cues are also used when we are teaching patients new skills as outlined in their plan of care. The only difference is that the prompts for the care plans are individual and are written in the patient's Adherence Improvement Plan (AIP). This cue (prompt) is to be used each time the program is run. Cues or instructions that we give family members or patients are to be given only one time. Do not repeat yourself. If you give a patient a cue or direction and he/she does not respond, use the prompting strategies described in the following pages.

This contrasts with the cues you will give patients outside of their AIP. These cues are not predefined or specified. However, prompts should not sound like orders like, "do this," "take this," etc. All cues or prompts should be delivered a pleasant tone of voice and should be friendly. For example, to get a patient to review their ileostomy care, you might say, "Hey Jim, let's go through the procedures for taking care of your ileostomy." Again, cues or instructions that we give to patients are given only one time. Do not repeat yourself. If you give your patient a cue or direction and that patient is hesitant, use the prompting strategies.

The behavior is just that, the behavior. It is the task or response that you get following your cue or prompt. Sometimes the behavior will be what you expect and what you asked a patient to do, and sometimes the behavior will not be what you asked.

The consequence is both the natural consequence of doing the behavior and the reinforcement you deliver for a patient's engagement in the correct behavior. It may be a social reinforcer or a quick trip to Starbucks. Regardless of the actual item delivered, remember that all reinforcement should include some verbal praise.

Remember, sometimes, family members or patients will not do what you ask or will not respond at all. You don't want to reinforce a patient for doing something other than when you ask (including not responding). So, what do you do then? Adherence Improvement Plan.

Key points:

- That the three components of instruction are:
- The antecedent (cue).
- The behavior.
- The consequence (reinforcement, punishment, penalty, extinction).

Now It's Your Turn:

- List one antecedent, one behavior that corresponds to that antecendent, and one consequence of that behavior.
- Look at your (or your patient's) care plan carefully. Highlight or underline all the specific instructions you (or your patient) is asked to do.

Prompting Strategies

There are people who can prompt others and be effective every time. Then there's the rest of us. Prompting is used to increase the likelihood that a patient will do a desired behavior. As behaviors are achieved, the prompting can be faded or reduced. In patient adherence, we are focusing on doing more of some behaviors (e.g., taking medications, exercising, and eating better).

There is also a fine line that is often crossed when people prompt to the point of annoyance. "Nagging," while it may initially sound like a prompt, is guaranteed to result in oppositional defiance and non-adherence.

Depending on the skills of patients, prompts can be verbal, gestural, or physical assistance to assist them in acquiring or engaging in adherent behaviors or skills. Prompts are generally given by a family member as a patient attempts to use a skill. It is important to remember that patients earn reinforcement as a part of protocols for the use of evidence-based adherence management practices. Thus, prompting strategies are foundational to the use of the evidence-based practices described in this book.

Full physical prompting (FPP) (e.g., shaping and molding the behavior with full touch and movement) will likely not be needed in most post-discharge patients with normally functioning physical abilities. FPP can be used effectively to address diabetic care when patients don't appear to understand verbal training.

Prompts are often categorized into a hierarchy from most intrusive to least intrusive.

Full physical assistance: The AdM Coach uses "hand-over-hand" support to aid the patient in completing a task (e.g., when teaching syringe filling, the AdM Coach make take the patient's hand and guides him with filling the syringe).

Partial physical assistance: The teacher provides partial physical assistance to help the child complete a task (e.g., when teaching the child to pick up the cup, the teacher guides the child's hand to the cup by tapping his elbow).

Full modeling: The AdM Coach models the desired behavior (e.g., The AdM Coach does each of the steps to syringe filling while describing it to the patient).

Partial modeling: The AdM Coach models only part of the desired behavior (e.g., when teaching how to fill an insulin syringe, the AdM Coach lays the materials out, but does not fill the syringe).

Full verbal prompts: The AdM Coach verbally models the desired behavior (e.g., when teaching the patient, the medical materials the AdM Coach asks him/her to name each of the materials).

Partial verbal prompts: The AdM Coach verbally describes only part of the desired behavior (e.g., when teaching the child to expressively label the insulin related materials, the AdM Coach asks, "What is this?").

Gestural prompt: The AdM Coach uses a physical gesture to encourage the desired behavior (e.g., when teaching the function of insulin related supplies and materials, the AdM Coach says, "Where is the insulin label?").

Not all the listed prompts need to be used for developing patient habits. Prompts should be chosen based on the learning needs of each patient. Prompts should be faded as quickly as possible to avoid prompt dependency. The goal of using prompts is to help patients become independent with their care.

Graphing

Graphs are our primary tool for displaying the data we collect. It can be challenging to determine if a patient's behavior is increasing or decreasing or if they are acquiring a new skill just by by looking at many individual daily sheets of paper. Graphs summarize data and give us the information needed to make decisions about adherence improvement.

A method we use to graph is the equal interval graph. This is the type of graphing you may have done in high school or college. There are seven components to this type of graph:

The X and Y-axis.

The vertical axis is called the Y-axis.

The horizontal axis is called the X-axis.

The y and the X-axis meet at the bottom left of the page.

Labels for the Y and X-axis.

The Y-axis tells you the behavior you are graphing. The Y-axis is where you would write the frequency or the duration of the behavior.

The X-axis tells you the units of time during which the behavior is recorded. This is typically in days, but it can be hours or minutes.

The numbers on the Y and X-axis.

There should be a hash mark on the X and Y axis to correspond to each of the numbers.

Data points.

Data points are plotted by locating the correct a unit of time on the X-axis finding the right unit of measurement on the Y-axis, and drawing a dot at the intersection of these two lines.

Data points must be graphed and correctly to indicate the level of behavior that occurred at each period.

Each data point is connected to the adjacent data points by a straight line.

Phase lines.

Phase lines are dashed vertical lines on a graph that indicate a change in treatment.

Data points are not connected across phase lines.

Phase labels.

Each phase in a graph must be labeled.

The phase label appears at the table of the graphs above the phase.

Title of the graph.

All graphs must be labeled using the title.

The title is a quick reference for what is displayed on the graphs.

Key points:

- Graphs are a tool to display data we collect and are used to make decisions about adherence.

Now It's Your Turn:

- Demonstrate how to plot data points on an existing graph.

Improvement Toward Adherence

The Adherence Improvement Plan (AIP) (See Appendix B for an example) is a tool that AdM Coaches use to document explicitly all the step-by-step things you will ask your patient to do in order to develop new adherence habits. You always follow the AIP as it is written. Never change the procedure as you Implement the AIP. That means, if a patient engages in any problem behavior, you do what the AIP states every time the problem behavior occurs.

The only person that can make changes to the AIP is your Advanced AdM Coach. The only time they would change or implement something that is not written in the AIP is after reviewing the changes with the primary care provider.

Planning Better Outcomes With The "Some Of The Time" Patients.

Better than 50% of the patient population has a history of non-adherence. Once these "at-risk" patients are identified using the B-MAAS/B-PAAS assessments, AdM Coaches determine why they are at-risk and what can be done to improve their behavior?

"I don't care how you get it done, just get it done." These words or similar words have long been used by healthcare providers and caregivers but have resulted in outcomes that were less than desired. People, in their role as patients, are still people. Teaching them to, "follow the plan of care" or do what the doctor wants them to do, has historically led to unsatisfactory outcomes. The most common statement coming that healthcare providers say regarding these non-adherent behaviors is, "what in the world were they thinking when they did, 'x'?" In any behavior improvement program, the desired behaviors must be stated in clear terms. Broad statements like, "Follow your discharge plan" are never sufficient.

Adherence Improvement Plan (AIP)

BEARS ADHERENCE IMPROVEMENT PLAN			
Patient Name:		Date:	
ID Number:	Diagnosis:		
AdM Coach:	Provider Name:		

The Adherence Improvement Plan (AIP) gives AdM Coaches©, patients, and family support groups an Applied Behavioral Approach to achieving better outcomes. The following sections review each area of the AIP to gain confidence in preparing a plan for patients you are responsible for. The first part includes demographics and is self-explanatory.

Can And Can't Reasons For Non-Adherence

In order to better understand the rest of the form, we will be looking at a particular HIV patient as described by Dr. Michael Stein. The completed form is attached in Appendix C. His patient's name is Beatriz (not actual name.) The first description demonstrates her non-adherence. "Beatriz's admission that she was missing pills was reasserted every three months. 'I forget, I don't keep them with me, she said."

When people "forget" to do the behaviors we need them to do to be adherent, it is always either a can't do or won't do situation. Your AdM Coach is tasked with determining whether your patient can't do (e.g., insufficient resources, doesn't have the skills or knowledge, etc.) or won't do the tasks to be adherent. Historically we assumed that if the patient wants to get "better" bad enough, they will do the required behaviors. If wanting anything "bad enough" was all that it took to become a world-class doctor or hockey player, then the world would be full of doctors and hockey players. There is a lot of sacrifices, and sweat involved with developing new skills and habits.

There are countless reasons patients will tell you why they "can't" follow their plan of care. For the most part, can't do reasons can be overcome by working with other members of the team such as social workers. First, we need to know the reasons why "at-risk" patients can't do a task. Determining the "can't do's" is very straight forward. The provided list are the most common excuses people have used for generations, to convince themselves and their clinicians why they can't be adherent.

AdM Coach:		Clinician Name:	
CARE PLAN CONSEQUENCE ANALYSIS REVIEW			
A1. Reasons I CAN'T follow my care plan		A2. Reasons I WON'T follow my care plan	
Rate	0-none, 1-A little, 2-Some, 3-A lot, 4-Intolerable	Rate	0-none, 1-A little, 2-Some, 3-A lot, 4-Intolerable
1	Inconvenience (not easily accessible)	3	Side effect of medications
4	Expense (Cost of medications)	0	Beliefs (religious restrictions)
1	Disability (Ability to be independent)	2	Defiance (Disgree with care plan)
1	Illness (Clinical restrictions)	1	Pain (Unable to do physical tasks)
0	Clinical complexity (steps and tasks)	1	Restrictions (Lifestyle change)
0	Time (Too many other requirements)	1	Route of Treatment (convenience)
3	Memory (Forgetful)	3	Culture (taboos or restrictions)
2	Storage for medical supplies	0	Inconsistent information (confusion)
	Other	0	Family disagrees with clinician (trust)
12	Subtotal	11	Subtotal
	12 of 32 38%		11 of 36 31%
Check	B1. I CAN follow my plan of care if...	Check	B2. I WILL follow my plan of care if my doctor...

Armed with the discharge or care plan, the BEARS Adherence Consequence Analysis (BACA) and the patient, the AdM Coach will go through each task in the plan and rate each from 0 to 4. After this exercise, Adherence Management Coaches will have an excellent picture of the whys patients can't follow their Care Plan. Beatriz told Dr. Stein that she "forgets" to take her pills. As a behaviorist and clinician, that statement tells me to look deeper into the "can't do" list for the root cause. For the most part, patients "can do" the adherent behavior if the "can't do" issues are resolved.

Houston... We Have A Solution

BEARS has provided a list of sample solutions in the "I CAN follow my care plan if..." to start the discussion with your patient once you have found out the "I can't" problems from the patient's perspective. If, for example, the primary issue is the cost of the medication, with the patient, you would have selected "Expense," and your patient might have selected 4-Intolerable.

Help me manage the cost of the medication, then the punishing effect (Negative, Immediate, Likely and Aware) will be removed. It does not guarantee your patient will take the drug, but it does ensure that the cost will no longer be a barrier or excuse to treatment. Eliminating barriers is an easier task and can be done relatively quickly. If you selected, "Is there a mechanism to manage out of pocket expenses?" Your case manager, social worker, AdM Coach© or other roles, should be familiar with the resources available in your community to overcome these barriers.

I Won't Follow Your Recommendations Doctor...

Dr. Stein continues, "We had established a lousy pattern. I would scold, and Beatriz would shrug or monosyllabically rationalize missing her pills. I was never sure what she was thinking."

As mentioned above, for every can't do, there is a possible and generally available solution. Non-adherent behavior based on can't do problems will almost always have a resource or training-based solution.

A. CARE PLAN CONSEQUENCE REVIEW					
A1. Reasons I "CAN"T" follow my Care Plan			A2. Reasons I ""WON"T" follow my CARE Plan		
Impact on Me			Impact on Me		
Write in Below	0-None; 1-A little; 2-Some; 3-A lot; 4-Intolerable		Write in Below	0-None; 1-A little; 2-Some; 3-A lot; 4-Intolerable	
3	Inconvenience (Not easily accessible)		4	Side effects of the medications	
5	Expense (Cost of Medication)		2	Beliefs (Religious objections)	
0	Disability (Ability to be independent)		5	Defiance (Disagree with care plan)	
2	Illness (Clinical restrictions)		0	Pain (Unable to do the tasks without pain)	
3	Distance (Transportation issues)		4	Restrictions (Lifestyle changes)	
1	Clinical Complexity (Confusing steps and tasks)		5	Culture (Taboos or restrictions)	
5	Time (Too many other requirements)		0	Inconsistent information (Confusion)	
4	Memory (forgetful)		3	Family disagrees with clinician (trust)	
0	Storage of medical supplies			Other:	
	Other:			Other:	

"Won't do" behaviors may be resolved through patient education and positive reinforcement, but often include firmly held beliefs by the patient that may be difficult to overcome. Won't do based on perceptions about the plan of care and the medications and their side effects can be managed through good patient education. Cultural beliefs offer an opportunity to understand why their feelings might interfere with the plan of care. These need to be understood, from the patient's perspective. Where changes can ethically be made, they need to be considered. Won't adhere to behaviors are generally good candidates for Motivational Interviewing and a non-confrontational examination of the beliefs.

Regardless of whether patients accept the plan of care and change their won't do to will, all behaviors in support of the plan of care should be heavily reinforced. The schedule of reinforcement can and should be thinned over time.

Moving Won't To Will… When You Can

Again, Dr. Stein, "She was missing so many doses that her virus was now dangerously out of control. I was exasperated with her. Getting her to change her behavior seemed hopeless and no longer worth the effort. This thought made me feel incompetent and empty and defeated."

Check Below	B1. I "CAN" follow my Care Plan if...	Check Below	B2. I "WILL" follow my CARE Plan if...
X	The prescription is more convenient with my schedule	X	My doctor can reduce or eliminate medication side effects
X	There is a way to manage my out-of-pocket costs	X	My doctor understands my beliefs about my illness
	Assistive devices can help my disability	X	My doctor understands my reasons for defiance
X	I can manage my care plan around my work		My doctor can manage my pain as a cause of nonadherence
	My provider is closer to my home or work	X	My doctor can evaluate and remove work/life restrictions
X	The clinical complexity of my care plan can be reduced		My doctor can find a convenient route of treatment
	The time requirements to do procedures is reduced	X	My doctor can identify and support my cultural differences
	Memory devices are available and easy to use		My doctor reviews and clarifies internet information
X	Medication storage is available and convenient		My doctor reviews and clarifies family information
	Other:		Other:

Once again, the responses as written in the "I will follow my care plan if…" section represents discussion points that AdM Coaches© can pick up on once the provider has made a referral for transition care. The AdM Coach© is specially trained to look at the consequences in the plan of care that contribute to patient non-adherence and come up with an alternative recommendation to share with the provider. Patient-centered care means the patient is involved in the decision-making process. Adherence Management Coaches© work through the plan of care with at-risk patients to get buy-in on the things the patient is willing to do. This feedback is then given to the provider and where accommodations can be made as appropriate. This adjusted plan of care is then shared with the patient and an Adherence Improvement Plan developed and implemented.

Pinpointing The Target Behavior

Results should be pinpointed first to avoid spending a lot of time reinforcing behaviors that do not result in the outcomes you are looking for in your patients. Specifically, ask yourself, "When will the outcome that I expect occur (e.g., lower B/P, decreased cholesterol, increased tolerance to exercise, etc.)? Outcomes are the product of behavior. List the Outcomes/Results in the column labeled "My Outcomes" (Column D1).

C. CLINICAL GOAL (WHAT DO I WANT TO ACHIEVE –e.g., better health, disease managed, etc.) Write in below"			
D. PINPOINT BEHAVIOR			
D1. My Outcomes/Results		D2. Behaviors Needed to Achieve Outcomes/Results	
What are the outcomes/results I can achieve by following my care plan?		What do I need to do (behaviors) to achieve improve health or wellness?	
1.	My viral load will be below 200	1.	I will take antiviral medications daily
2.		2.	I will record my time on my AIP graph
3.		3.	
4.		4.	
5.		5.	
6.		6.	
7.		7.	

Behavior pinpoints are not thoughts, feelings, attitudes or beliefs. They are neither internal, subjective, nor abstract. Cognitive-behavioral terms such as improve motivation, increase morale, ensure communication, and establish rapport all sound like worthy "behaviors." They require pinpointing because each may represent a series of behaviors. Adherence is made up of many behaviors and often, we use labels as a shortcut rather than describe the target behavior. There is nothing wrong with saying that a "patient is cooperative." When your AdM Coach writes in the Adherence Improvement Plan that the "patient will cooperate with his/her clinician," what are the behaviors associated with "cooperate?" These specific behaviors will be written in the "Patient Behavior" column (Column D2).

Your AdM Coach will keep the following points in mind when writing "behaviors":

Patients must have control of the behavior

Behaviors are active

Measure for effectiveness

E. MEASURE BEHAVIOR			
E1. Patient Centered Outcomes/Results		E2. Behaviors Needed to Measure the Outcomes/Results	
How will if know if my behavior is improving my health?		How will I measure my behavior in following my care plan?	
1.	My viral load will be below 200	1.	I will take antiviral medications daily
2.		2.	I will record my time on my AIP graph
3.		3.	
4.		4.	
5.		5.	
6.		6.	
7.		7.	

The idea of measuring behavior, and charting or developing graphs to show progress may seem to be a chore or waste of time. In many instances, this belief is the result of a history of having charts used as a form of punishment. For most of our lives, charts, graphs and other measurement products have been used as a "do-it-or-else" tool. In applied behavior, our graphs are used to celebrate achievement. Even small steps in the right direction are celebrated. Many people might say, "why celebrate the little steps, anyone can do that?" The simple answer is that behavior change requires a nudge. Momentum is created when doing the right thing is celebrated. Using the measuring chart as a tool for reinforcement encourages more use of the tool. When patients (people) see their graph moving in a right direction, the graph itself becomes a reinforcer.

Key points:

- Measuring reduces emotionalism.
- Measuring increases credibility for clinicians in support of their plan.
- Measuring demonstrates progress or the lack of progress.
- Progress requires measurement.
- Progress offers opportunities for celebration.
- Measurement points to the behaviors to achieve progress.
- Results are what's leftover when the response is done.

Whose Job Is It Anyway?

Dr. Stein continues with his story, "I asked Beatriz who knew about her test results. No one except her husband, she said… she wanted to keep it that way … She hadn't told her sister… She hadn't told her mother…She hadn't told her best friend… If anyone found out about her HIV, there would be humiliation, guilt, embarrassment."

F1. How will my Outcomes/Results be Measured?			F2. Who will measure my behavior?		
Check List		Tally Sheet	Self monitor		Pharmacist
Graph		Calendar	Family member		Nurse
Other			Nurse		Other
How often will my outcomes/results be measured?			How often will my behavior be measured?		
Daily	Weekly	Monthly	Daily	Weekly	Monthly

Managing a chronic illness is a team effort. The bottom line is that if we want to move the bar in favor of "persistence," it will take more than one 15-minute appointment with their provider every three months to provide adequate reinforcement.

New habits, as Mark Twain once wrote, "Habit is habit and not to be flung out of the window by any man, but coaxed downstairs a step at a time." It impossible, with a patient load of 2,000 souls, to be at everyone's stairwell three times a day to reinforce the new habits. This is a family responsibility.

The question is, who will measure the outcomes and the behavior? Dr. Stein needed help in managing his frustration with Beatriz. Out of sight is out of mind and as he wrote in this piece, "I had cared for thousands of HIV patients like Beatriz."

Adherence Improvement Plan (AIP) Page Two

Dr. Stein's dilemma, "There was a risk of family's fear, blame, unkind words, the possibility of withdrawal, and a refusal or unwillingness to help. While Beatriz might find some support, she didn't expect any. Beatriz turned down my suggestion to speak to a counselor, as this would mean the revelation of her secret to another person, and I was concerned about her isolation."

Reinforcing The Target Behaviors

People will not do behaviors that don't have some kind of payback or reward for doing them. Most adherence improvement programs focus on antecedents or the tasks necessary to get the patient to do things at least once. AdM Coaching focuses on reinforcing the target behavior when it occurs to promote it occurring again. The list of antecedents can be very long or quite short. The illness itself is an antecedent. Antecedents serve as cues for behavior. Without illness, it is not likely that patients would stop their day-to-day activities to drop into a clinic. Prescriptions are cues for obtaining medications. Headaches are an antecedent for looking for aspirin, getting a glass of water and taking the pill. Pill bottles, blister packs, buzzers, and an almost endless list of things serve as antecedents for adherent behavior. If they were effective, then there would be no patient non-adherence in the world today. Antecedents also become a part of the background noise related to everyday living. Some antecedents will get our attention some of the time but not all of the time.

Positive Reinforcement.

What happens after a desired behavior that can increase the likelihood of that behavior becoming a habit? Positive reinforcement is the answer. Many people have the idea that reinforcement is the same as bribery. In reality, there is a world of difference. "If patients get something good for nothing, then patients will become good for nothing." Bribery is getting something (a reward), ahead of time, for doing nothing at the time of the reward. There may be the promise of "going to exercise, going to start a diet, going to take my pills," but too frequently, the reinforcer is given, and no behavior is given in exchange for the bribe.

Reinforcement is an "If-then" deal with your patient. "If you take your medications as prescribed for a week, then you can have a free massage in the clinic." Always remember the famous words of the late President Ronald Reagan, "Trust but verify."

Positive reinforcement is the best way to get patients on the straight and narrow path to adherence. You need a plan, and the plan needs to be followed. The single biggest problem with medication adherence is that there is little or nothing positively reinforcing about taking a handful of pills. The consequences of pill taking behavior are clinically POSITIVE or good for the patient. The POSITIVE nature of the consequence is weakened because it occurs sometime in the FUTURE. It is equally important to remember that, while the outcome of the medication is LIKELY, patients are frequently NOT AWARE of the consequences. From a perception level, consequences with a POSITIVE-FUTURE-LIKELY-NOT AWARE profile are as if the consequence never happened at all. Behavior that is NOT positively reinforced with something POSITIVE-IMMEDIATE-LIKELY-AWARE or the behavior is ignored altogether (extinction.), the behavior will eventually stop. Knowing that to be the case, then the AIP is used to develop a schedule that reinforces the patient's behavior. The most potent reinforcers are those that have a POSITIVE-IMMEDIATE-LIKELY-AWARE profile. From the patient's perspective, this profile lets them know their behavior has a consequence; the consequence is good for them; the consequence is good for them while they are doing the target behavior; the consequence is good for them every time they do the behavior, and they are aware that they were positively reinforced. If all medication prescriptions had this profile, non-adherence would end tomorrow.

Since that is not the case, we must plan to reinforce adherent behavior.

H. BEHAVIOR REINFORCEMENT PLAN		
Plan for reinforcing my Behavior		
Baseline		
Final Goal		
H1. My Behavior subgoals:		H2. How will my Behavior be Reinforced?:
1.		1.
2.		2.
3.		3.
4.		4.
5.		5.
6.		6.
7.		7.
G		G

Your Reinforcement Plan allows us to work with patients to define the outcomes we believe are essential. For example, if the result is maintaining an A1C level below 6%, in the row labeled Baseline, we would write in the baseline or starting A1C level. In this example, we will use 8.5% and consider the patient to have poor diabetes management. Our Final Goal might be maintaining an A1C level at or below 6. Behavior Sub-Goal Dates can be quarterly checks to ensure we are on task and can be done just before the patient visiting the doctor. Why before the visit? We want to celebrate patient outcomes and that can be with the whole treatment team. The Celebrate Dates should be written into your patient's AIP.

Why do we determine the Outcomes before identifying the behaviors? Knowing where the patient is going (outcomes) sets the course for the behaviors necessary to reach their goals. Once again, we look at the Baseline and write in what is being done today. It describes the behaviors that need to be done to achieve the Final Goal. Typical behaviors may include diet and exercise. What are your current baselines? Where would you like the behaviors to be to achieve the goals. The AIP provides space to set your goal dates and then celebration dates. How you plan to celebrate and the reinforcers available to your patients can be determined by completing the Reinforcer Survey.

Getting The Behavior Started And Maintaining It

Dr. Stein tried using antecedents to promote adherence. "She had tried setting an alarm to remember her evening dose. I thought of engaging her husband…"

Care plans do not establish healthy habits. They merely suggest what habits need to be created. The best way to get a habit started is to ensure that behavior is positively reinforced. Most of the habits people have are a result of those behaviors being reinforced enough times to become habit.

The problem with taking medications is they offer little or no immediate feedback or reinforcement. They simply work, especially in the long term. On the other hand, the costs, side effects, scheduling, etc. are all immediately punishing. When new behaviors are needed, they must be reinforced heavily initially and then the reinforcement schedule can be thinned. If no one is responsible for identifying antecedents in the plan of care and consequences are not planned to reinforce the target behaviors, then all behavior will return to baseline. Baseline, when it comes to people, is not taking medications. For the most part, people will spend 40 or more years without having to pay attention to their health or take medications to prevent a worsening of a medical condition.

Getting Patients On Board

I. ADHERENCE PLANNED ACTIVITIES					
I1. Planned antecedents for implementing my care plan			I2: Planned activities for providing feedback to me		
Who	Does what	When	Who	Does what	When

In order to help your patient to "Buy-In" to the Adherence Management Plan, antecedents ("patient behavioral cues") must be considered carefully and designed skillfully if patients are to change their behavior. Setting the conditions for change to occur is a crucial behavior AdM Coaches need to master. Antecedent management, along with consequences, provides the clarity needed for achieving adherence. Patients and their families may not have the skills necessary to identify these factors without guidance.

Many clinicians consider the use of reminders as antecedents without understanding their limited power to maintain desired behavior. Careful planning in initiating healthcare strategies is also important to healthcare success. Clinicians and AdM Coaches should not neglect the attention that antecedents deserve as powerful triggering events.

Antecedents are any events that come before a behavior, in this case, taking prescribed medication(s) and provide information about the consequences. Planned antecedents can be as simple as filling a weekly pill container or setting the alarm or buzzer to remind the patient it's time to take a pill. Write the name of who is going to fill the pill container, "Who," "Does What," and "When" (on Sunday evening or whenever). Each of the steps needs to be considered and written in this area. Pill bottles can't be filled if there are no pills in the house. Who (does what) is going to pick up the prescription? When do they need to do it? Every behavior has a series of steps that need to be considered. Each of these must be added to the list.

Behaviors are typically associated with many antecedents and consequences. They seldom are random actions. Antecedents can get a behavior started or added to the repertoire of many behaviors we all go through every day. It's the consequences that keep the behaviors going or cause them to stop. Behaviors that are repeated enough times and have positive reinforcement, become habits. Our goal in Adherence Management Coaching is to achieve habit levels when it comes to following a plan of care.

A. CARE PLAN CONSEQUENCE REVIEW					
A1. Reasons I "CAN"T" follow my Care Plan			A2. Reasons I ""WON'T" follow my CARE Plan		
Impact on Me			Impact on Me		
Write in Below	0-None; 1-A little; 2-Some; 3-A lot; 4-Intolerable		Write in Below	0-None; 1-A little; 2-Some; 3-A lot; 4-Intolerable	
	Inconvenience (Not easily accessible)			Side effects of the medications	
	Expense (Cost of Medication)			Beliefs (Religious objections)	
	Disability (Ability to be independent)			Defiance (Disagree with care plan)	
	Illness (Clinical restrictions)			Pain (Unable to do the tasks without pain)	
	Distance (Transportation issues)			Restrictions (Lifestyle changes)	
	Clinical Complexity (Confusing steps and tasks)			Culture (Taboos or restrictions)	
	Time (Too many other requirements)			Inconsistent information (Confusion)	
	Memory (forgetful)			Family disagrees with clinician (trust)	
	Storage of medical supplies			Other:	
	Other:			Other:	

Medication taking behavior will have at least two sets of consequences. The first consequence is automatic. If the pill is taken it will likely do what it was developed for. The problem with this is that many medications work below the perception threshold.

Thousands of patients have told their clinicians that they quit taking their medication because they couldn't feel any difference.

On the other hand, others have stopped taking their medications because they get a negative consequence such as side effects. Side effects should be reported to the prescribing provider as soon as possible. The other set of outcomes is a little more planned. The fastest way to a new habit is through positive reinforcement. Consequences that are positive, immediate, certain and are valued by the patient need to be paired with the desired behavior. Who is going to do what (provide reinforcement) and when? Reinforcement works best when it is provided immediately after the target behavior. A list of reinforcers can be developed and used when the behavior is completed.

The difference between AdM Coaching© and other adherence improvement programs is the emphasis on identifying punishing elements in the plan of care and opportunities to reinforce the plan over time. Remember: Antecedents start behavior. Consequences maintain behavior. The two operating together establish the most reliable conditions for individual and healthcare success. Adherence Improvement Plans are nothing more than an antecedent for improving adherence. Consequences such as positive reinforcement increases the likelihood of patients following their care plan.

Key points:

- An Adherence Improvement Plan (Appendix B1 and B2) is the tool AdM Coaches use to document explicitly what needs to be done to develop and strengthen new adherent habits.

- Always follow the Adherence Improvement Plan as written.

- Do not change any procedures in the Adherence Improvement Plan. Only the clinical director or Advanced AdM Coach can change the plan.

- Implement the Adherence Improvement Plan as written.

- Procedures in the Adherence Improvement Plan should be followed every time medication or wellness behaviors occur.

Now It's Your Turn:

- Make a copy of a blank AIP.

- Fill out as much as you can as an exercise. Bring it to your next primary care visit to discuss ways you or your patient can become more adherent.

AdM Home Coach Professionalism

Responsibilities of an AdM Home Coaches are listed in the various sections of this book. In addition, you are to;

Follow the directions on each patient's Adherence Improvement Plan (AIP) for adherent behaviors and skill development and each time a problem behavior occurs.

Collect data as assigned.

Record and chart data as assigned.

Train other caregivers as required.

Also, when you first start your daily routines as the patient's caregiver, do the following:

Talk with the any other AdM Home Coach, who was working with the patient to learn the current status of your patient and his/her progress. If you cannot talk with the AdM Home Coaches, read the AdM Coach notes.

Gather reinforcers or potential reinforcers you may need for the shift. Remember, you should always know what reinforcers are used and their effectiveness. Have them ready to use when the behavior occurs.

Maintain any documentation, including the ABC narrative, and training worksheet (See Appendix I.)

Key points:

- It is essential to follow the Adherence Improvement Plan and to record each time adherent behaviors and problem behaviors occur.
- You are responsible for collecting data as assigned.
- You are responsible for charting data as assigned.

Now It's Your Turn:

- Use a blank sheet of paper and start collecting data about a specific behavior that you or your patient does on a regular basis. For example, record with tally marks every time you (or your patient) washes their hands per day. Do this for two days.
- At the end of two days, make a chart with Day 1 and Day 2 on the X-axis. And the number of times washed on the Y-axis (make sure

you write increment marks such as 1,2,3… or 2,4,6…) so you can quickly compare the two days.

Your Emotions

Even though you may be self-confident and good at doing your job, you also need to be aware of your own feelings and emotions as you interact with your patient. You must be able to control them to be active with patients. Working as an AdM Home Coach can be stressful and hard work. It can be frustrating and at the same time rewarding. You'll have adherent days and non-adherent days with your patient. It is how you react and handle these non-adherent days that play a significant role in your interactions.

When you are having a bad day because of something personal in your life (something outside the patient's environment), you need to do your best to leave this issue outside. You may be agitated, irritated, or angry. These are all-natural emotions, but it is how we handle these emotions that is important. When you are angry, fearful, tired or anxious, patients may recognize these and typically, it may cause an increase in problem behaviors.

Also, when you're having a bad day, you may not feel like supporting the care plan, so you decide you are going to let the patient do whatever they want and you're not going to do anything about it. This too will reinforce more problem behaviors and not just on your bad day, but also in the future. Remember new habits need consistency. A lack of consistency will increase the likelihood of returning to old habits.

When you have days like this, try to remain as calm as possible and non-reactive. Do not let your emotions show in your speech or your body language.

How Patients Interact With You.

How family members, in their role as a patient, will communicate with you depends much on your behavior. If you have a positive attitude towards them and their disease is being managed, family members will be more cooperative.

How family members interact with you can also depend on a few other factors. First, their physical condition or health can impact how they interact with others. How do you interact with others when you have a headache? Typically, you do not respond or interact positively. Patients are the same.

Second, the environment that they are in can also have an impact. If the situation is disorganized, patients may become less adherent. If they are confined in any way, it may led to having cabin fever and increase non-adherence.

A third factor is a patient's ability to communicate. If family members are communicating effectively, they will tend to have fewer non-adherent behaviors. Also, if family members are being rewarded for their communication, that is reinforcement, patients also tend to have less non-adherent behavior. The patient's physical limitations, medications, and other illnesses can also affect how they react.

Although several factors are influencing how to apply the AIP, remember the most critical factor is you and your behavior.

Key points:

- How we interact with family members who are our patient can be a positive strategy in adherence management.
- Building relationships with your patient can improve adherent behavior.
- Building relationships takes time and effort on your part.
- To build relationships, deliver both contingent and non-contingent reinforcement.
- Reinforcement is an excellent tool for establishing adherent behavior.

- Be sure to have a "time-in" that is filled with a reinforcer, interaction, and attention.

- Give patients choices.

- Patients who have choices are typically more cooperative and motivated.

- Giving choices gives them a sense of control in their own lives.

- Your self-confidence plays a role in how you interact with patients and how they interact with you.

- If you're not confident in your skills and are afraid of your patient, they will sense it, and it may cause more problem behavior.

- Be aware of your emotions when working with patients.

- If you're having a bad day before you see the patient each day, leave it outside.

- When you're having a bad day, you need to continue your work and interact with your patient as if you weren't having a bad day.

- The patient's interaction with you may depend on their physical condition, health, environmental factors, and their ability to communicate.

Now It's Your Turn:

- List some ways you can leave your bad emotions outside.

- List some ways you can stay positive throughout your interactions with your patient.

What Do I Do If My Patient Is Not Cooperative?

There will be times when your family member/patient is not cooperative. That is, he or she is not following your directions and not doing what you ask. Remember that not following instructions is considered a non-adherent behavior or an inappropriate behavior because it is something you don't want to happen again. When a family member is not cooperative, there are some things you can do to try and get them to cooperate. The most effective method is typically changing the reinforcer you are using.

Typically, if they are not cooperating with their AIP, they are not being properly reinforced. Remember that people behave as they do to get something or to avoid doing something. So, if a family member is not going along with their care plan, he/she typically does not know what he/she is going to get out of it. Remember that reinforcers can change from moment to moment; that is, what is reinforcing right now may not be reinforcing in 10 minutes.

In either case, you need to look at the reinforcer you are using and change it because it is no longer working as a reinforcer. So how do you change it? Remember the strategies for figuring out what is reinforcing. You can see when your patient is not going forward with their care plan. You can give your patient a choice of reinforcers. Regardless of what method you use to figure out what the reinforcer is now, the critical thing to remember is that changing the reinforcer can increase compliance cooperation.

Key points:

- If family members are not cooperating, he or she is not being properly reinforced.
- Find reinforcers that will motivate your patient by changing from one reinforcer to another, or giving your patient a choice of reinforcers.
- Uses the strategies listed above to see what is motivating your patient at that moment.

Now It's Your Turn:

- List four reinforcers that your patient wants.

What Do I Do When My Family Member Or Patient Engages In Adherent Behavior?

How we respond to our family member's adherent behavior will determine how they act in the future. Remember, adherent behaviors are those behaviors that we want to happen again or more often in the future. How do we increase the behavior? We use the procedures of reinforcement.

When patients engage in an adherent behavior, reemember to reinforce it. You can give the patient an item, object, or activity they like, and socially praise them. Remember, each time you provide an object or action as a reinforcement, always pair it with social praise.

When a family member engages in adherent behavior, never ignore it. If you ignore adherent behavior, patients will be less likely to engage in that behavior in the future. Therefore, you must recognize adherent behavior no matter how small it may seem to you.

When family members follow directions, this is adherent behavior. Reward It!

Key points:

- When family members engage in adherent behavior, always reinforce it.

- Always pair items, objects, or activity of reinforcers with praise.

- Never ignore adherent behavior.

- Ignoring adherent behavior will make it disappear.

Now It's Your Turn:

- List two adherent behaviors (actions) and two praises for those actions.

What Do I Do If What A Family Member Is Engaging In Non-Adherent Behavior?

When patients engage in non-adherent behavior or inappropriate behavior, then never reinforce it. Do not provide a patient with any attention, praise, or any reinforcing item for the non-adherent behavior. A rule that applies to all non-adherent behaviors is that you want to minimize all reinforcement, as much as possible.

When a behavior is reinforced, we increase the likelihood of its occurrence in the future. Since non-adherent behavior is not desired, do not reinforce it and remove any and all reinforcement that may be occurring naturally. Reinforcing non-adherent behavior will increase that action, and that is why we stress minimizing support each time it occurs.

You may not realize you're reinforcing your patient for non-adherent behavior. Your AdM Coach may give you feedback about reinforcing non-adherent behavior or show you how to handle the behavior in the future. Be sure to listen carefully to their explanations as they are trying to help improve your skills and ultimately to improve the clinical outcome.

Key points:

- Never reinforce non-adherent behavior.
- Reinforcing behavior increases its occurrence in the future.
- Often families will reinforce non-adherent behavior, and they don't mean to or don't even know that you are reinforcing it.

Now It's Your Turn:

- List two non-adherent behaviors (actions).

Stop-Redirect-Reinforce Technique.

Sometimes patients engage in non-adherent behavior that may not be listed explicitly in the AIP. So, what do you do then? One method is the stop-redirect-reinforce technique.

The first step in this technique is to stop the non-adherent behavior from recurring. This may mean blocking the patient from engaging in the problem behavior while providing as little reinforcement is possible.

The second step is to redirect the patient to another activity or by instructing that he or she can comply. This task is not to be a strongly reinforcing task or behavior. This step is crucial to the procedures because you want a family member to engage in tasks that you can reinforce and by redirecting them, you're presenting a job for them to complete — using prompting if necessary to get the patient to complete the job.

Once the patient has completed the task or followed your direction, you reinforce this behavior by providing social praise, an item, object, or other activity. Although you deliver reinforcement, you do not reinforce actively or heavily.

Key points:

- Use the stop-redirect-reinforce technique for non-adherent behaviors.

- First, stop the non-adherent behavior from occurring.

- Second, redirect the patient to another activity or by giving an instruction (this should not be a reinforcing activity for the patient) — prompt the patient engaging in the task if necessary.

- Third, reinforce patient to engage in this new activity or task but not heavily.

Evaluating When You Get Stuck

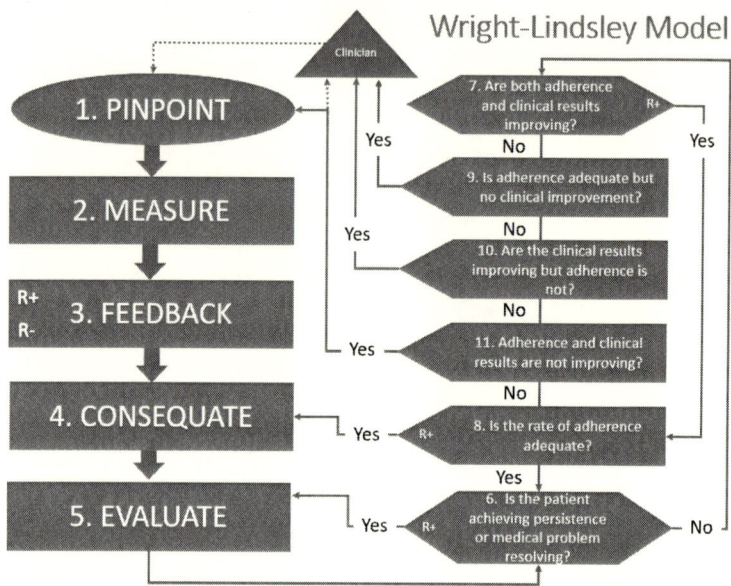

Who You Gonna Call? Every AdM Home Coach© is going to run into family members or patients that test their ability to work with them. With 7 billion people on the planet and thousands of variables, not including their illness, you have to fall back on your AdM Coaching training to find solutions to adherence problems.

With every patient, whether family member or no relation, you need to ask the question, "Am I making a difference? Are we achieving persistence (long term adherence habits)?" The Wright-Lindsley Model (See Appendix F) provides a roadmap from beginning behaviors to persistence habits.

AdM Home Coaches are focused on behavioral change. You may feel challenged, because of experience or training, to get inside your patient's head and deal with their "cognitive dissonance" or ambivalence. You may feel inclined to push or pull them through each of the steps associated with pre-contemplation to maintenance and relapse prevention.

AdM Home Coaches do not need to have advanced degrees in psychology, counseling or social work to effectively work with changing a family member's behavior. Pinpointing elements in the plan of care should be identified in terms of observable behaviors rather than some internal conflict due to previous experiences. If AdM Home Coaches© had to deal first with ambivalence or wrong thinking, how long would it take for family members to become adherent? Probably forever.

The causes of non-adherence are mostly external (e.g., cost, inconvenience, side-effects). The AdM Coach transition team fills out the Adherence Improvement Plan, which focuses on identifying "punishers" in the care plan and removing or modifying these punishers with the patient and their clinicians. They pinpoint the results that the patient or family member needs to achieve and the behaviors necessary to achieve those results.

Then, with the AIP in hand, you as the AdM Home Coach, can begin to look for and identify those behaviors that achieve those correct results. You measure a baseline and share it with the patient. You and your transition care team establish a reinforcement plan. As new behaviors are recorded, you consequate those behaviors as appropriate, and then evaluate the patient's progress, starting daily, then weekly, monthly, quarterly (Steps 1 through 5).

Once you get comfortable with your ability to measure and reward adherent behaviors, you will move into the next phase to determine if all your efforts are paying off. You start to ask yourself, "Is the patient achieving persistence? Are adherence goals and clinical results improving? Is the rate of adherence adequate? and most importantly, do we need to get further help from our healthcare provider or clinician?"

As you walk through these questions, you can make assessments of your reinforcers. Are they effective? Do they need to be changed? Am I reinforcing enough or should I thin out the schedule to achieve persistence?

Common Reasons Adherence Fails

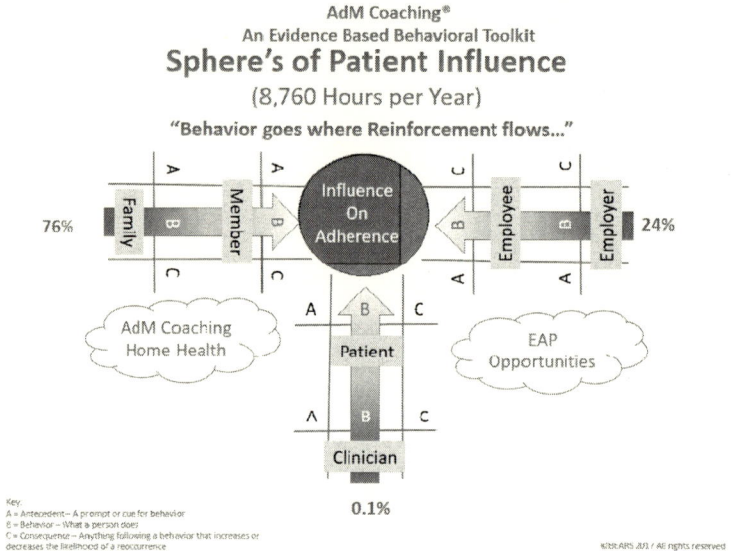

Beyond the health care system, Applied Behavioral Analysis (ABA) has been used successfully over the past thirty-five years and refined through the efforts of Dr. Aubrey Daniels under the titles "performance management" and "behavior-based safety." Thousands of people have enjoyed his training programs and developed expertise over the years.

The success or failure of any adherence plan depends upon who the patient is listening to and where they are getting their information. The graphic on the previous page provides an overview of the three major con-tributors or influencers of patients as they begin their new care plans. While the literature supports the notion that physicians may be the best patient educators, both patient load and length of clinical visits between patient follow-up rule against any consistency of purpose or sufficiency of positive reinforcement to improve adherence to create habits.

The historical reality that even Hippocrates wrote about non-adherent patients, a couple of thousand years ago, attests to the fact that people are going to do what is most reinforcing for them. Time with face-to-face clinician encounters is often less than four hours per year, which accounts for less than 1% of the total number of hours that a patient spends in one year.

The next highest patient support center, which may also be a source of conflicting information, is found in the patient's place of work. There are increasing opportunities for other people to present incorrect medication information or leading patient decisions through anecdotal details about other employee's experiences with medications or treatment plans.

Dr. Ivar Lovaas' warning, "without positive reinforcement, all behavior returns to baseline" is a reminder that not taking pills is a person's usual baseline. So, when they have to start taking pills two, three, or four times a day without internal and external sources of reinforcement, at least half of all patients will "return to baseline" and stop following their care plan.

Large employers may want to consider offering formal Employee Assistance Programs (EAPs) that include Adherence Management Programs to support the needs of employees with chronic health care needs. The employer-based Adherence Management Coach provides an opportunity to work with patients who find it difficult to follow their care plan, especially at work. As AdM Coaches, these occupational health nurses could prove to be a valuable source for identifying "at-risk" employees and implementing their care plans over the time of their employment. People are typically at their workplaces 2,080 hours per year.

Lastly, the biggest influencer is the time a patient will spend with family and friends at home. There are more than 6,000 hours with the people who have a real investment in their relationship with the patient. These are the people who, when the consequences of non-adherence occur, are left behind to pick up the pieces. When handed a care plan and perhaps a few minutes of pointing out critical parts of the plan; and, when the door closes at the clinic or hospital and opens at home, the family member becomes the only source of positive reinforcement. You are the "home caregivers" but lacking the experience and training to understand what is essential to bring out the best results from your patient's care plan.

How Adherence Management Might Let You Down.

There are clearly defined causes why adherence management programs might not achieve your goals. This information is courtesy of the many years of Dr. Daniels' experience. The following list is in no particular order. What matters is that unless measures and adjustments are made to correct for them, a combination of factors assures the failure of any behavior change initiative.

Limiting Your Care Plan Commitment.

The best example of limiting commitment begins in the hospital or care facility with discharge training. I have frequently heard transitional care nurses state, "I don't have time for training the patient. I'm responsible for ensuring their O2 concentrator, wheelchair, walkers, and so forth arrive at their home." Another often-heard phrase is, "Have you seen my workload? This place loads me down with nine or ten admissions per day and another five or six discharges."

Transitional care nurses don't know which patients are at risk for non-adherence, have not explored the care plan consequences, from the patient's perspective, and have no idea how to develop and implement an Adherence Improvement Plan (AIP) with patients or their families. Patients and their families often leave the acute care setting in a fog of confusion with a bag full of orders, prescriptions, educational materials, and follow-up appointments with only a vague idea of how to implement them.

Care plan commitment begins by creating new habits. But, new habits are seldom the first thought a patient or caregiver has when questions arise at home. Pinpointing the desired outcomes and defining the behaviors necessary to achieve those results needs to be the first step. This is done in the AIP.

The following questions need to be explored before patients, and their families leave the hospital, acute care, or long-term care facility. What training is needed? Are the necessary resources available? Is there enough time to do the task? How will we reinforce the target behavior? What is reinforcing for each of the participants? Do we have the necessary reinforcers available?

Not Believing The Behavioral Process Is Evidence-Based.

"What you are asking us to do is just common sense." This is the quickest response when people are satisfied with the status quo or do not want to invest their time, effort, and resources in improving their health outcomes. Throughout history, people have spent minimal effort in maintaining their health until something goes wrong. Now they have to focus on resource-intense health concerns. When they don't achieve their expectations within a few days or weeks, medical science and their care plan must have failed them. The reality is they failed the science. "Did you educate the patient?" is the most frequent question I hear daily from insurance payers and state agencies. If they were "educated properly," then we expect them to perform. Payers want patient adherence and they want it now! Incorrect behaviors can be stopped immediately, given enough punishers. But creating new habits will take coaching and reinforcing.

Beyond believing in the effectiveness of applied behavior, are the consequences built into care plans. The desired results (improved health and reduction of illness) are often months or years away, while the immediate results (inconvenience, side effect, confusion, distrust, and acceptance) are present now. Immediacy affects patient behavior as they "choose" to abandon their care plan. Evidence-based results (creating new habits) means that people, on both sides of the care plan, must understand that consequences affect adherence.

No Investment In Coaching To Yield Habit-Strength.

Every long-term health benefit has a cost. The question is, is the benefit worth the price? Will the change reduce expenses or improve clinical outcomes? Aristotle (384BC – 322BC) recognized that we are what we do. "Excellence, therefore, is not an act but a habit. We are what we repeatedly do." Dr. Ivar Lovaas (1927 – 2010) correctly stated that all behavior returns to baseline. A baseline is any behavior that preexisted before the care plan was written. It is the old habit that may have been around for years. Dr. Aubrey Daniels, in a private conversation with me, stated clearly, "Our job is to change the baseline." How are baselines changed? Provide positive reinforcement for the desired behavior, long enough to make it a new habit. Reinforce the desired behavior frequently and then thin the schedule over time. Behavior goes where reinforcement flows. Stopping reinforcement too early guarantees a return to the non-adherent baseline. Providing intermittent reinforcement for the new behavior ensures the new habit will continue and become the new baseline. What are the costs associated with long-term health improvements? Time and money.

I Thought An Introduction To Behavior Would Solve My Patient's Problems.

An introduction is just that—an opportunity to look into The Science of Behavior for a chance to understand better. An introduction is never enough for any patient adherence effort. The same holds true for Teachback efforts, Motivational Interviewing, Medication Therapy Management, and the various other initiatives through the decades that have failed to significantly improve patient adherence.

It requires a commitment to learning, implementing, and maintaining your understanding of The Science of Behavior. The quickest path to returning to the old ways (e.g., smoking, overeating, and no exercise) is to understand that punishment and penalty may stop these behaviors today.

Without replacing life-long habits and reinforcing desired behaviors, old habits return over time. Adherence improvement efforts are short-lived if patients return to their old ways of doing things once their new actions are no longer reinforced.

Lost track of antecedents and consequences and how they are used.

A primary issue with adherence programs today is losing track of antecedents and reinforcers when implementing an adherence improvement plan. You may know the behavior you are seeking, but if you don't know how to cue that behavior and you are not aware of consequences that strengthen and increase that behavior, it is unlikely you will get the results you want. All behaviors, whether we recognize them or not, have cues (antecedents) and consequences. Not all cues lead to behavior, but consequences always strengthen or weaken target behaviors. One other thing is abundantly clear when working with patients; what is reinforcing for one person can be punishing to another. Items that are effective cues in one environment may be readily overlooked in another. Knowing which antecedents are useful in what environment for which patient, and then appropriately reinforcing the desired behaviors when they occur are essential to measure and record.

No Accountability Was Established.

There is an old adage in healthcare that if you didn't write it down, you didn't do it. We like to think we are consistent in recognizing the accomplishments of our employees. Then I hear, "I thought Jill would do it." "I didn't know that that was my job." "I'm not the boss of her." Accountability is the issue. Health service delivery is becoming increasingly complicated. The topography frequently changes. What used to be acute care is now skilled home care. What was skilled home care is now a family responsibility. Implementing a behavior-based program requires families to have more than a cursory understanding of The Science of Behavior and how to apply it.

The Adherence Improvement Plan identifies the roles of AdM Home Coaches, patients, and clinicians. Family coaches and other members of the team have accountable functions that are identified and supported.

Lifestyles Didn't Change… Did Not Incorporate R+.

When family members become part of the Adherence Management team, they need to know that it requires a lifestyle change in the way they interact with the family member/patient. The caregiver becomes the primary reinforcer of adherent behaviors. Not adapting to meet this new or updated challenge is often insufficient to effect behavioral change in your patient. It is also insufficient to expect clinicians to provide enough positive reinforcement to effect change. When clinicians are asked how reinforcing they are, most will generally say either they are, or they could be better. When family members are asked about their provider as being reinforcing, most will tell you they get very little support from their provider in the way of reinforcement. A simple measurement tool is this. If a provider feels they are positively reinforcing their patients, they probably are not. Feeling that you provide positive reinforcement and documenting the types, intensities, frequencies, recording the results of those R+s are two very different things.

Past performance is always the best indicator of future performance. As home caregivers, we too, often return to old living habits because we have not learned how The Science of Behavior works. As an AdM Home Coach, we must not only provide positive reinforcers (R+) but also document the type, frequency, intensity and results of these consequences to ensure lasting change in our patient. No consequences for supporting or not supporting the care plan process will result in care plan abandonment.

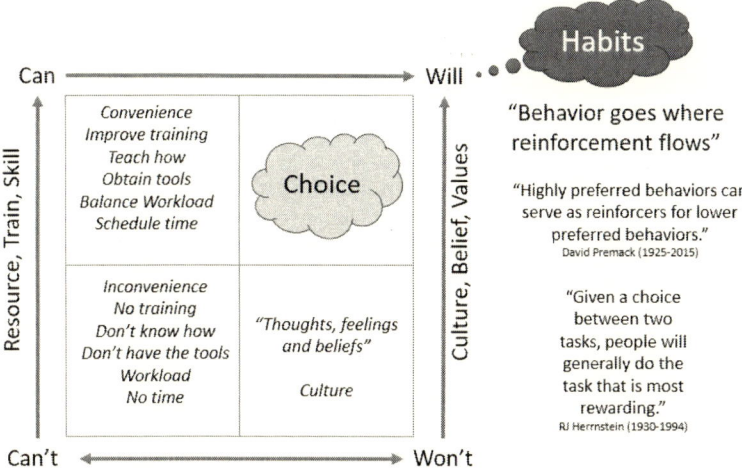

New care plans are often surrounded by some start-up fanfare and then quickly become part of the day-to-day background noise.

The life-as-usual culture re-emerges, and another innovative care plan bites the dust. "Consequences" have taken on the appearance of something foreboding. Perhaps the 1960s TV show "Truth or Consequences" may have helped set the stage for the misinformation about the truth of consequences. Your answer was either the truth, or you faced the consequences. Culturally the term consequence has always taken on a dark definition. "If you don't do as told, you'll suffer the consequences." Every behavior has a consequence. Positive consequences are those we enjoy and repeat. Negative consequences fall into two categories: penalty, or losing something that we have and want, or punishment, getting something that we don't want. We live in a rule-governed society and implementing rules should be a regular part of consumer behavior. The initial thought of consequences for most people is, "We need to punish people who interfere with the program."

It is almost an institutional observation that punishment is the natural consequence of not following the rules. In applied behavior, reinforcing desired behavior is the preferred consequence for developing new skills. ABA accepts that target behaviors are shaped. Incremental improvement is reinforced, and punishment for not meeting a target is ignored (where appropriate). Penalty stops undesired, as well as desired behavior. Equally important is understanding that extinction or ignoring behavior will end both wanted and unwanted outcomes. Extinction is a consequence where all behavior-based functions go to die.

The following is not a strict ratio, but a general principle in Applied Behavioral Analysis. Reinforcers should be used at least four times more often for the desired behavior than punishment or penalty is applied for undesired ones. This ratio does not mean that you offer four reinforcers and then you need to punish undesired behavior. What is created by focusing on reinforcement is a positive culture. Many health services facilities could learn from this rule. Frequently, I see nurse leaders overlook the many great efforts of staff nurses or even patients, and then punish the occasional mistake. If your family member is improving in their behavior, be quick to reinforce that behavior also if the behavior is not quite right.

Shaping, correcting, and reinforcing is the fastest way of creating new habits. Penalty and punishment represent the quickest path to non-adherence, making excuses, covering mistakes, and lies.

No Investment In Training Home Based Coaches.

How many times will hospital patient educators say, "Read this book, you are now the home expert on following your care plan."?

Change requires commitment, and commitment is a human resource. How well are patients and their families trained on the day of discharge? What level of competence is s/he working? Is the family AdM Home Coach invested in implementing their care plan? Does s/he have a working knowledge of the science, and do they support the patient and want to work with their hospital counterpart AdM Coach? Are the family and patient supportive of behavior change? AdM Home Coaches must understand The Science of Behavior, see the benefits related to this approach and become advocates. When family members and patients provide only cursory support, another opportunity arises to demonstrate that applied behavior coaching is ineffective, if not applied at all levels – from hospital to home.

Thought That Education Alone Would Improve Adherence.

The most common response regarding patient adherence when management is not happy with unplanned readmissions is to say they (e.g., patients, staff educators, or transitional care nurses) need more education. In many instances, training has become a new way of counseling staff members on their performance. It avoids the time-consuming factors of establishing whether or not the staff member or patient can't do or won't do the needed work. Retrain the staff, have them all sign the training slip. Then we can hold them accountable when behavioral change does not occur. The question is, "Will training correct 'won't do' behaviors?" The answer is, "No!" When staff is tasked with multiple tasks, not related to training, then there is not a focus on ensuring staff has the skills they need.

Thought They Knew More Than What 80+ Years Of Research Has Confirmed.

There have been many fads regarding organizational improvement over the past several decades (See chart below Business Fads). Organizations have spent millions, if not billions, on motivational programs and process improvement systems only to discover disappointment down the road when applied to human behavior.

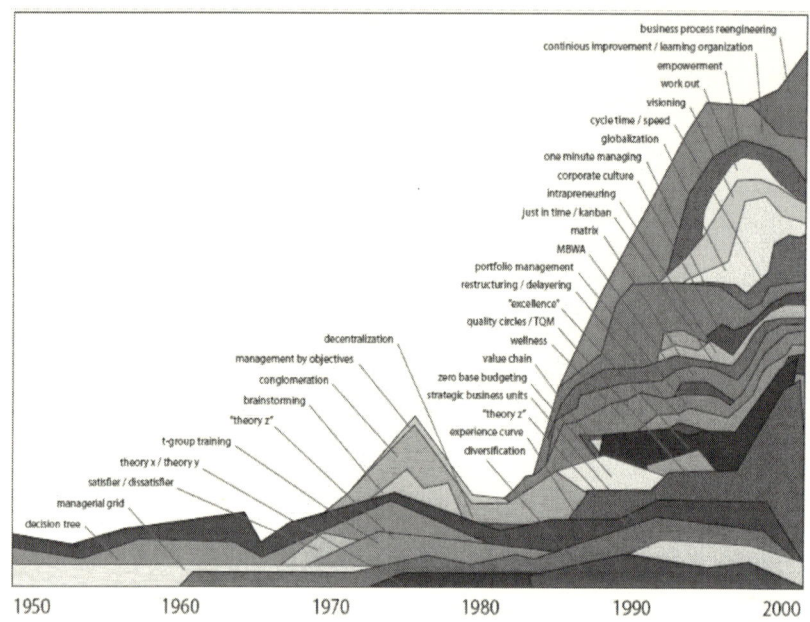

Improving systems without understanding the consequences for people implementing them is filled with peril. Adherence improvement is about behavior change and creating new habits. So why review some "business fads?" Health services programs are notorious for tapping into the business world and taking business process improvement programs and evolving them into health care improvement programs.

While these adaptations reduce the time needed to develop the next new thing, their focus is on improving health services delivery processes and not changing patient behavior.

Fad based behavior changes, such as empowerment (introduced in the late 1980s), have not moved the needle on adherence. Some significant patient education efforts and medication therapy management, as well as motivational programs, are persistent. However, since their focus is on antecedent cueing of behavior, they have not made the expected changes in behavior. The past eight decades of applied behavior science has evolved through developing skills and ending self-injurious habits with children and adults on the autism spectrum. More than four decades ago, Dr. Aubrey

Daniels furthered the scientific application by introducing Performance Management into human behavior in the workplace arena. From performance, he further looked at and expanded the role of applied behavior into behavior-based safety. As we entered the second decade of the 21st Century, this author extends the applied research into health care. Following care plans means doing more of some behaviors and less of others. We need more adherence to medication, dietary, and exercise regimens and less smoking, drinking, and overeating.

Epilogue:
The AdM Home Coach Beginning

Significant strides have been made in improving the health care system and reducing harm to patients while they are in the hospital or long-term skilled nursing facilities. But little progress has been made to improve long-term adherence after the patient leaves these facilities. The key to any behavior change is to get and sustain people's interest in developing new and healthy habits. We need to invite families into the conversation between nurses who are trained in Adherence Management Coaching and improvements to patient follow-up care programs. There are significant negative consequences associated with patients who are unwilling to learn how to improve their health through following their care plan.

BEARS Adherence Improvement Plan (AIP) makes following discharge and care plans meaningful to patients. It is used to engage family members and patients in the change process from old unhealthy habits to new healthy ones. By getting behaviorally involved, patients and their families become stakeholders in adherence advocacy and medication persistence.

AdM Coaches are putting non-adherence issues out there for all to see. The fact that over 125,000 people die each year because they choose not to follow their plan of care is staggering. If there are other programs out there that are successful, why are so many people struggling with adherence? Adherence Management Coaching (using Applied Behavior Analysis techniques) is the solution for developing long-term, habit-forming, persistence in following medical advice. For at least the last 35 years, cognitive approaches (thoughts, feelings, and beliefs), patient education (Teachback), and antecedent manipulation (changing pill bottles, creating new labels, pill-minders, and timers) have been tried again and again. The results are not impressive. The patient change that needs to take place is behavior-based. Every family wants their medically affected family member to follow their care plan. For 80% of patients with a chronic and manageable disease, they still choose not to follow medical advice. It is the consequences of adherence that often lead to care plan abandonment (e.g., inconvenience, confusion, expense, and side-effects). Manage the consequences, create and reinforce new habits, and adherence will improve.

There is an old Vietnamese saying we can learn from, "A thousand hearings is worth one seeing and a thousand 'seeings' is worth one doing." We have all heard the statement, "If I told them once, I told them a thousand times." A thousand hearings will not change behavior. Seeing and hearing are not behaviors. There is nothing to reinforce. Only when there is a 'doing' that can be counted, shaped, strengthened; and, given enough doings and enough reinforcement for doing, can we create a habit. Creating adherent habits is the function of the AdM Home Care Coaches.

Improving Patient Safety is Behavior-Based, Too!

The behaviors of patients, visitors, nurses, chaplains, aides, and countless others result in 19,000 people dying each year from Methicillin-Resistant Staphylococcus Aureus (MRSA), and 100,000 people will have extended stays in hospitals for treating their hospital-acquired MRSA. When people are asked how this could happen, the response is often, "It's a hospital, what do you expect? It is just what happens when you put sick people together. It comes with the territory."

Does this statement make inadequate patient safety excusable? Can healthcare staff members say, "It's just the way it is," and then abandon their patient safety programs? What are the behaviors of non-compliance? Many plagues have started with cross-contamination from poor hand hygiene. Individuals, patients, staff, caregivers, and family members must all become aware that healthy, persistent habits save lives and healthcare costs.

There are health systems in place at the hospital or care facility levels that are beyond a patient's control. These are the hospital improvement initiatives that use Six Sigma or LEAN to improve processes and procedures as they relate to medical professions and patient safety. In contrast, their programs focus on improving operations, but not the behaviors necessary to achieve adherence. BEARS behavior improvement programs focus on strengthening behaviors and enhancing patient and staff safety to ensure patient and employee behaviors do not defeat better process initiatives.

To learn more about AdM Coaching or to take the NEXT STEP into telehealth and certification, join us at www.admcoaches.com/homebundle.

Appendix

Appendix A1:
BEARS Adherence Consequence Analysis (BACA)

Consequence Analysis for Plan of Care

Patient's name:	Jean Doe		Current Problem:	Post AMI with Stent
Date:	3/15/2016	Medications:	Clinician:	Jane Doe, MD

The following information is my evaluation of the consequences of following or not following my provider's recommended plan of care. I have reviewed the consequences from my perspective and have recorded them by placing an "x" in the blocks below.

Plan of Care/Post AMI Stent placement

ANTECEDENTS	BEHAVIOR	CONSEQUENCES	P	N	I	F	L	U	A	N
	Choose to **not take** medication as Prescribed									

	BEHAVIOR	CONSEQUENCES	P	N	I	F	L	U	A	N
	Take medication as Prescribed									

(P) Positive = good for me;
(N) Negative = not good for me

(I) Immediate = during the behavior;
(F) Future = some time later

(L) Likely = consequence may happen;
(U) Unlikely = consequence may not happen

(A) Aware = I can perceive the consequence,
(N) Not aware I will not perceive the consequence

Appendix A2:
BACA SAMPLE

Consequence Analysis for Plan of Care

| Patient's name: | Jean Doe | | Current Problem: | | Post AMI with Stent |
| Date: 3/15/2016 | Medications: | Effient 20mg | Clinician: | | Jane Doe, MD |

The following information is my evaluation of the consequences of following or not following my provider's recommended plan of care. I have reviewed the consequences from my perspective and have recorded them by placing an "x" in the blocks below.

Plan of Care/Post AMI Stent placement

ANTECEDENTS	BEHAVIOR	CONSEQUENCES	P	N	I	F	L	U	A	N
Family history of heart disease	Choose to **not take** Effient as Prescribed	AMI		x		x		x	x	
Spouse concerned		Death		x		x		x	x	
Friend died from AMI		Heart disease		x		x	x		x	
Had a heart attack		No side effects	x		x			x	x	
Had chest pain		Chest pain		x	x			x	x	
Shortness of breath		Reduced activity		x		x		x	x	
Lightheaded		Short of breath		x	x			x	x	
Had stents placed		Save money	x		x		x		x	
Family worried	**Take Effient as** Prescribed	Cost		x		x	x		x	
Fear of death		Bruising		x	x			x	x	
Fear of lost work		Reduce AMI risks	x			x		x	x	
Stent(s) placed		Pill Schedule	x		x			x	x	
Retire early		Tired feeling		x	x			x	x	
Cardiac cripple		Live longer	x			x	x		x	
Children complain		Reduced AMI risks	x			x		x	x	
		Nausea		x	x			x	x	

(P) Positive = good for me;
(N) Negative = not good for me

(I) Immediate = during the behavior
(F) Future = some time later

(L) Likely = consequence may happen;
(U) Unlikely = consequence may not happen

(A) Aware = I can perceive the consequence;
(N) Not aware I will not perceive the consequence

Appendix B1: Adherence Improvement Plan (AIP) Page 1 Of 2

BEARS' ADHERENCE IMPROVEMENT PLAN				
Patient Name:				Date:
ID Number:			Diagnosis:	
AdM Coach:			Clinician Name:	

CARE PLAN CONSEQUENCE ANALYSIS REVIEW				
A1. Reasons I CAN'T follow my care plan			**A2. Reasons I WON'T follow my care plan**	
Rate	0-none, 1- A little, 2- Some, 3- A lot, 4- Intolerable		Rate	0-none, 1- A little, 2- Some, 3- A lot, 4- Intolerable
0	Inconvenience (not easily accessible)		0	Side effect of medications
0	Expense (Cost of medications)		0	Beliefs (religious restrictions)
0	Disability (Ability to be independent)		0	Defiance (Disgree with care plan)
0	Illness (Clinical restrictions)		0	Pain (Unable to do physical tasks)
0	Clinical complexity (steps and tasks)		0	Restrictions (Lifestyle change)
0	Time (Too many other requirements)		0	Route of Treatment (convenience)
0	Memory (Forgetful)		0	Culture (taboos or restrictions)
0	Storage for medical supplies		0	Inconsistent information (confusion)
0	Other		0	Family disagrees with clinician (trust)
0	Subtotal		0	Subtotal
0 of 32		0%	0 of 36	0%
Check	B1. I CAN follow my plan of care if...		Check	B2. I WILL follow my plan of care if my doctor...
	The prescription is convenient with my schedule			can eliminate or reduce side effects
	There is a way to manage out of pocket costs			understands my beliefs about illness
	Assistive devices can help my disability			can manage my pain as a reason for non-adherence
	I can manage my plan around my work			can evaluate and remove work/life restrictions
	My provider is closer to home or work			can find a convenient route of treatment
	The complexity of my plan can be reduced			knows and supports my cultural values
	The time to do procedures is reduced			reviews and clarifies internet information
	Memory devices are available to use			reviews and clarifies family information
	Medication storage is available and convenient			Understands my reasons for non-adherence

C. CLINICAL GOAL (What I want to achieve: better health, disease managed, etc.) Write in Below:

D. PINPOINT	
D1. My Outcomes/Results	**D2. Behaviors Needed to Achieve Outcomes/Results**
What are the outcomes or results that I can achieve by following my plan of care?	What do I need to do (behaviors) to have better health wellness?

D1. My Outcomes/Results		D2. Behaviors Needed to Achieve Outcomes/Results	
1		1	
2		2	
3		3	
4		4	
5		5	
6		6	
7		7	

E. MEASURE BEHAVIOR	
E1. Patient Centered Outcomes/Results	**E2. Behaviors Needed to Measure Outcomes/Results**
How will you know your behavior is improving health?	How will you measure your behavior to follow your plan of care?
1		1	
2		2	

Appendix B2:
Adherence Improvement
Plan (AIP) Page 2 Of 2

F1. How will Outcomes/Results be measured?		F2. Who will measure behavior?	
Check list	Tally sheet	Self-monitor	Pharmacist
Graph	Calendar	Family member	Social Worker
Other		Nurse	Other

How often will Outcomes/Results be measured?			How often should behavior be measured?		
Daily	Weekly	Monthly	Daily	Weekly	Monthly

G. RESULTS REINFORCEMENT PLAN
Reinforcement Plan for Outcomes/Results

Baseline	
Final Goal	

G1. Results subgoals:		G2. How we will Reinforce Results:
1.	1.	
2.	2.	
3.	3.	
4.	4.	
5.	5.	
6.	6.	
7.	7.	
G	G	

H. BEHAVIOR REINFORCEMENT PLAN
Plan for reinforcing Behavior

Baseline	
Final Goal	

H1. Behavior subgoals:		H2. How we will Reinforce Behavior:
1.	1.	
2.	2.	
3.	3.	
4.	4.	
5.	5.	
6.	6.	
7.	7.	
G	G	

I. CARE PLAN ACTIVITIES

I1. Planed antecedents for implementing Care Plan			I2. Planned activities for reinforcing Behavior		
Who	Does what	When	Who	Does what	When

Appendix C1:
Baca For Beatriz.

BEARS Targeted Adherence Consequence Analysis for Plan of Care

Patient Name	Beatriz		Target Behavior:	Take Prescobix 1 time daily
Date:	06/11/2016	Provider prescribing plan of care	Dr. Stein	
AdM Coach©	R. Wright, PhD, RN			

ANTECEDENTS	BEHAVIOR	CONSEQUENCES	P	N	I	F	L	U	A	N
Diagnosed with HIV		Her doctor disappointed with her		X		X			X	X
Fear of death		HIV out of control		X		X	X			X
Family worried	What may	Disease gains power		X		X		X		X
Fear of lost work	happen if I *don't*	Disease grow stronger		X		X		X		X
Fear of disability	*follow* the Target	Medication loses potency		X		X		X		X
May lose job	Behavior	Run out of treatment options		X		X	X		X	
	described above?	No medication side effects	X		X		X		X	
		No cost for medications	X		X		X		X	
		Schedule not restricted by medications	X		X		X		X	
		Dr. may drop her from practice		X		X		X	X	
		Spouse nags patient to take pills		X	X			X	X	

ANTECEDENTS	BEHAVIOR	CONSEQUENCES	P	N	I	F	L	U	A	N
Visit to Drs. Office		May cause liver damage		X		X		X		X
Diagnosis		Liver damage is life threatening		X		X		X		X
Prescription		Severe life threatening skin reactions		X		X		X		X
Teachback		Can cause kidney failure with meds		X		X		X		X
Counseling	What may	Diarrhea, mouth sores, tiredness		X		X		X		X
Disease symptoms	happen if I *follow*	Nausea, fever, muscle and joint pain		X		X		X		X
Spouse nagging	the Target	High blood sugar		X		X		X		X
	Behavior	Diabetes or worsening diabetes		X		X		X		X
	described above?	Increased bleeding in hemophilia		X		X		X		X
		Changes in body fat		X		X		X		X
		Two medications in one pill	X		X			X		X
		Cost $1,862.12 per month		X	X			X	X	
		High genetic barrier to resistance	X			X		X		X

ANTECEDENTS	BEHAVIOR	CONSEQUENCES	P	N	I	F	L	U	A	N
Fear of the unknown		New counselor will know information		X	X		X		X	
Visit to Drs. Office		May lose mother		X	X		X		X	
Diagnosis	Disclose illness	May lose sister		X	X		X		X	
Prescription	and seek	May lose friends		X	X		X		X	
Teachback	counseling	Will cause shame		X	X		X		X	
Counseling		Fatalism (This is meant to be)		X	X		X		X	
Beliefs		Husband engaged with family	X		X		X		X	

Plan of Care/HIV diagnosis

		Strongest to Weakest Consequences								Extinction Consequences							
Consequences →		PILA	NILA	PIUA	NIUA	PFLA	NFLA	PFUA	NFUA	PILN	NILN	PIUN	NIUN	PFLN	NFLN	PFUN	NFUN
		Most Power		Upper Middle		Lower Middle		Least Power		Least Weakness		Upper Middle		Lower Middle		Most Weakness	
Behavior(s)																	
Non-Adherent		3	1				1		2						1		3
Adherent		6	3		3										3		
Disclose illness		1	6														

NFUN – Consequences the patient is not aware of represent "extinction" events. Regardless of how good or bad the consequence is, if your patient is not aware that the consequence is occurring, then it is as if the consequence never happened at all. Any behavior that is put on extinction will stop. They key to the NFUN is that you are asking the patient to do something today (e.g., take a pill). If she does not, the consequences are FUTURE and UNLIKELY. Something bad might happen, but not today or the near future. As her viral load increases, she will be largely unaware that it is occurring. She may have symptoms of diarrhea, but not today. The concept of immediacy should never be underestimated. If I buy these medications, the cost will affect me in a NEGATIVE way today. Spending money on medications is an IMMEDIATE event. NEGATIVE, IMMEDIATE, LIKELY and AWARE events will frequently stop adherent behavior. Beatriz has three NILA consequences for being adherent. These may be sufficient to overcome PILA's that are available for her. The essential task in developing her Adherence Improvement Plan is finding ways to weaken the NILAs. Sharing information about her HIV presents as a very punishing event and needs to be addressed to increase her support based and people who can provide her with positive reinforcement between office visits with Dr. Stein.

Patient's Signature		AdM Coach's Signature	

Appendix C2:
AIP For Beatriz

BEARS' ADHERENCE IMPROVEMENT PLAN					
Patient Name:	Beatriz 1234			Date:	4/3/2017
ID Number:	12345		Diagnosis:	HIV/AIDS	
AdM Coach:	R Wright, PhD., MHA, MA, RN		Clinician Name:	Dr. M. Stein	
CARE PLAN CONSEQUENCE ANALYSIS REVIEW					

A1. Reasons I CAN'T follow my care plan		A2. Reasons I WON'T follow my care plan	
Rate 0-none, 1- A little, 2- Some, 3- A lot, 4- Intolerable		Rate 0-none, 1- A little, 2- Some, 3- A lot, 4- Intolerable	
4	Inconvenience (not easily accessible)	2	Side effect of medications
4	Expense (Cost of medications)	4	Beliefs (religious restrictions)
0	Disability (Ability to be independent)	3	Defiance (Disgree with care plan)
0	Illness (Clinical restrictions)	0	Pain (Unable to do physical tasks)
0	Clinical complexity (steps and tasks)	4	Restrictions (Lifestyle change)
4	Time (Too many other requirements)	0	Route of Treatment (convenience)
0	Memory (Forgetful)	4	Culture (taboos or restrictions)
0	Storage for medical supplies	3	Inconsistent information (confusion)
0	Other	0	Family disagrees with clinician (trust)
12	Subtotal	20	Subtotal
12 of 32	38%	20 of 36	56%

Check	B1. I CAN follow my plan of care if...	Check	B2. I WILL follow my plan of care if my do...
X	The prescription is convenient with my schedule	X	can eliminate or reduce side effects
X	There is a way to manage out of pocket costs	X	understands my beliefs about illness
	Assistive devices can help my disability		can manage my pain as a reason for non-adhere
	I can manage my plan around my work		can evaluate and remove work/life restrictions
	My provider is closer to home or work		can find a convenient route of treatment
	The complexity of my plan can be reduced		knows and supports my cultural values
	The time to do procedures is reduced	X	reviews and clarifies internet information
	Memory devices are available to use		reviews and clarifies family information
	Medication storage is available and convenient	X	Understands my reasons for non-adherence

C. CLINICAL GOAL (What I want to achieve: better health, disease managed, etc.) Write in Below:
I WILL TAKE MY MEDICATIONS EACH DAY AS PRESCRIBED BY MY PHYSICIAN

D. PINPOINT	
D1. My Outcomes/Results	D2. Behaviors Needed to Achieve Outcomes/Results
What are the outcomes or results that I can achieve by following my plan of care?	What do I need to do (behaviors) to have better health wellness?

	D1		D2
1		1	
2		2	
3		3	
4		4	
5		5	
6		6	
7		7	

E. MEASURE BEHAVIOR	
E1. Patient Centered Outcomes/Results	E2. Behaviors Needed to Measure Outcomes/Results
How will you know your behavior is improving health?	How will you measure your behavior to follow your plan of care?
1	1
2	2

Appendix D:
Dr. Wright's Evaluation Of
"Losing Control."[3]

"I kept trying to come up with new memory devices to help her improve pill-taking, hoping that it was simple forgetfulness."

These thoughts played like a stuck record for Dr. Michael Stein as he worried over Beatriz. She had not followed her HIV plan of care for more than three years. Dr. Stein wrote of his efforts in educating Beatriz, setting up pill minders, and doing a seemingly endless array of tasks to overcome her ambivalence. To his extreme frustration, nothing worked. These "common sense" approaches did little to help her understand that not sticking with her plan of care would result in increased suffering and an early trip to the grave. Education and motivation had no impact on her behavior. What she did after leaving his office was up to her. The negative consequences of years to come in not following her care plan had little sway over the negative consequences she faced every day in following her plan.

Nothing is more easily forgotten than taking a handful of pills day after day. I am sure you have noticed that things people enjoy doing rarely end up in that pile of unfinished tasks at the end of each day. To be sure, there are times that things are forgotten and then picked up at the next opportunity, but what is reinforcing about taking pills?

---

3   Stein, Michael, (2016) Losing Control, Harvard Review. Accessed online https://www.harvardreview.org/content/losing-control/. The author highly recommends reading Dr. Stein's article. Non-adherence affects everyone. Dr. Stein reveals the frustration physicians also face with their non-adherent patients.

Forgetfulness Is A Symptom Of Negative Consequences.

"Beatriz's admission that she was missing pills was reasserted every three months. "I forget. I don't keep them with me," she said. I warned her at every visit that forgetting to take her pills two or three days a week would get her in trouble..." Dr. Stein wrote, "I needed her to be perfect with her pills."

There were 129,600 minutes between office visits and then 15 minutes with Dr. Stein. For Beatriz, these 15 minutes of cajoling, praying, hoping, explaining, teaching, and frustration were surrounded by 129, 585 minutes of little or no positive reinforcement. How much impact can a clinician have when their contribution to life, living and reinforcing the care plan is only 0.0001%? Can "...perfection with her pills" reasonably be expected when competing signals are present 99.999% of the time? Inconvenience may occur 2 or 3 or more times every time she stops to take medications. Side effects may occur from time to time or perhaps with every pill she takes. Co-pays are faced at least three times between visits and choices must be made between feeding her family, paying the rent and slowing down the relentless process of chronic disease. "I needed her to be perfect..." but then, Dr. Stein needs all his patients to be perfect and the most perfectly adherent patient is the one in the exam room now. Between the present appointment for Beatriz and the next, Dr. Stein will likely see 1,920 patients. In a practice focusing on HIV/AIDS patients, all will need to be perfect. Statistically, 230 will not fill their prescriptions. An additional 230 will fill the prescription and put it in on the shelf. Five-hundred fifty-seven will, like Beatriz, inconsistently take their medications. Finally, nine-hundred twenty-one will stick to their plan of care

BEARS Has A Plan For You

To achieve adherence, as well as you can, you need to identify the consequences that are punishing adherent behavior. Consequences come in many forms. BEARS reviewed the research of many agencies and divided the results into an easy mnemonic: ICE-IF-SAD (Inconvenience, Choice, Expense, Illness, Forgetful, Side Effects, Accepting, and Distrust). While almost 70% of non-adherence is attributed to behavior, the only choice is a behavior. Choice is the linchpin in the formula because choice is a function of convenience, expense, illness, side effects, acceptance and distrust. Patients choose to take or not take their medications because of the consequences. "Simple forgetfulness" is a passive explanation of choice. Perhaps your patient forgot to take his or her medicines because the cost was too high or the side effects too many. Forgetfulness is not a behavior. I often refer to it as a "bridge excuse." It fills the time when clinicians ask why they didn't take their medications and the often-used response, Behaviors are always based on the consequences of following a plan of care. Knowing why your patient chose to forget or chose not to fill the prescription is a step towards making your plan of care more patient-centered. When patients forget, you need to search for why. The answers are always in the consequences.

Care Plan Punishment

People avoid punishing consequences. Whether they get something they don't want (punishment) or avoid the loss of something they have and want (penalty), negative consequences are something normal people avoid. Particularly sick ones.

Few providers think of their care plans as punishing. Punishment violates the 2,000 year-old Hippocratic admonitions to "first do no harm." From the provider's perspective, care plans offer just the opposite. Harm refers to injury or damage and is easily overlooked when the pharmacopeia describes the treatment as improving, reducing or stopping harm. At the same time, all providers are aware that many medications have side effects. Some medication therapies once started, will be lifelong commitments to a daily regimen of care. Both consequences, from the patient's perspective, are punishing.

Health care journals are full of articles listing the value of being "patient-centered." The 2010 National Healthcare Disparities Report stated there is a need, "To provide all patients with the best possible care, providers must be able to understand patients' health care needs and preferences and communicate clearly with patients about their care."

Today it is not enough to know your patients are nonadherent. We need to understand why they are nonadherent. How can you possibly address their behavioral issue when you don't know where the problem lies? BEARS' offers a quickly learned tool kit that can be used with the patient to assist you in looking at the "punishers" from the patient's perspective.

Beatriz, You Need To Do This…
Show Me Why You Can't.

Patient centeredness goes beyond just doing the right thing for the patient. It goes beyond providing educational materials. It also includes identifying the things your patients are likely not to do. Everything we ask outpatients to do have Positive and Negative consequences. Also, the consequences can be either Immediate or Future, Likely To Occur or Unlikely, and your patient may be either Aware or Not Aware of the Consequences. Going through the care plan with the patient using the BEARS Consequence Analysis is the most patient-centered way to achieve adherence and persistence. There is power in the consequences. Consequences that are Positive, Immediate, Certain, and the patient is Aware of the event are highly likely to improve adherence. Conversely, Negative, Immediate, Certain and Awareness of the consequences will stop adherence.

I am reminded of the inscription on the James Farley Post Office in New York City that reads, "Neither snow nor rain nor heat nor gloom of night stays these couriers from the swift completion of their appointed rounds." This inscription was not based on the US Postal Service, but rather the mounted couriers of Persia in 500 BC. It showed that all things could be endured when the consequences of the behavior are positively reinforced. It is possible to improve adherence such that patients let neither inconvenience, nor expense, nor illness, nor forgetfulness, nor side effects, nor distrust stays them from the appropriate implementation of their plan of care.

Process, Performance, Or Adherence Management.

For many decades, the search for improved patient outcomes has focused on managing processes. "Drive out errors" was the cry. Improve the process, and the quality will follow. No doubt this is true. Out of this recognition came TQM and Six Sigma, to name a couple. What of human error? Improve performance and quality will follow. The result of this thinking was Performance Management and the use of applied behavioral science. Where this has been consistently applied, the results have been remarkable. For at least the last half-century, when it comes to patient behavior, the focus has been on education and motivation. "Teach them and they will comply." "Overcome their ambivalence and they will comply." When these approaches failed to make significant gains in Hospital Engagement Network (HEN) 1.0 the recommendation was more emphasis on patient education. After HEN 2.0, the advice was to reduce the standard down by 5%. Adherence Management requires an applied behavioral solution. "Wrong-thinking" and ambivalence management have a role but changing behavior focuses on providing positive reinforcement to both achieve adherence and develop persistence.

Appendix E:
Reinforcer Survey

REINFORCER SURVEY TOOL

NAME		Date:				AdM Coach:			
			Category			Reinforcer Type		A Little	A fair amount	Much	Very Much
	Reinforcing Activities	P	J	S	T	S2	1	2	3	4
1.	Spending time with hobbies		X							
2.	Surfing trip	X								
3.	Water Skiing trip			X						
4.	Sailing trip		X							
5.	Listening to music	X								
6.	Classical music	X								
7.	Easy listening	X								
8.	Listening to Jazz	X								
9.	Watching sports	X								
10.	Watching Adventure movies	X								
11.	Watching War movies	X								
12.	Watching Musicals	X								
13.	Playing Sports			X						
14.	Watching TV	X								
15.	Watching Fox News	X								
16.	Watching Discovery Channel	X								
17.	Attending parties and/or events			X						
18.	Being with Friends			X						
19.	Attending Community organizations			X						
20.	Participating in Outdoor activities		X							
21.	Watching video games		X							
22.	Completing a difficult job			X						
23.	Singing	X								
24.	Dancing	X								
25.	Spending Time with family	X								
26.	Playing an instrument			X						
27.	Shopping			X						
28.	Playing cards with friends	X								
29.	Spending Time with friends	X								
30.	Being around other people	X								
31.	Involvement with church/mosque/temple			X						
32.	Writing blogs	X								
33.	Relaxing under a tree	X								
34.	Parenting			X		X				
35.	Cooking for friends			X		X				
36.	Playing video games	X			X					
37	Praise for achieving goal(s)			X						
38.	Asking my opinion			X						
39.	Free coffee and doughnuts	X								
40	Time with my clinician	X								

P = Pleasure; J = Joy; S = Satisfaction; T = Tangible; S2 = Social

Appendix F:
Wright-Lindsley Review Process

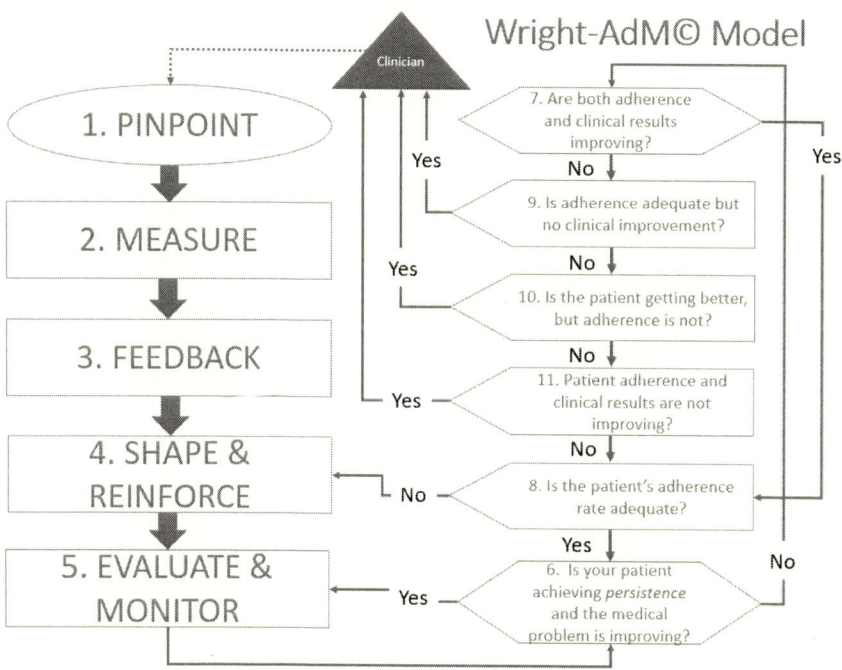

Appendix G1:
BEARS' Medical Adherence Assessment Scale (B-MAAS)

Behavioral – Medication Adherence Assessment Scale (B-MAAS)				
Date Assessment Completed:			Total Score:	
Name:			Risk	
Reviewer:				
Select 1 Level per category based on your assessment and write in the score 0 through 3	**0**	**1**	**2**	**3**
1 Married	Yes	No		
2 Gender	Female	Male	Low Risk 0-12 / Mild Risk 13-24 / Medium Risk 25-36 / High Risk >37	
3 Motivated to improve health/condition	Yes	No		
4 Ethnicity	Caucasian	Non-Caucasian		
5 Education	College	High School	Middle School	Elementary
6 Age	>80	60-79	40-59	20-49
Vision Impaired	No	Mild	Medium	Severe
8 Hearing Impaired	No	Mild	Medium	Severe
9 Memory Impaired	No	Mild	Medium	Severe
10 Intentional defiance	No	Mild	Medium	Severe
11 Patient/Provider Relationship	>7 visits	5-7	2-4	0-1
12 Medication Side Effects Present	No	Mild	Medium	Severe
13 Family Income	High	Medium	Low	None
14 Physical Disability	No	Mild	Medium	Severe
15 Disease Symptoms Present	Severe	Moderate	Mild	No
16 Mental illness Diagnosis/Dementia	No	Mild	Medium	Severe
17 Attitude About Recovery	Good	Moderate	Fair	Bad
18 Understands Disease	Yes	Some	Very little	No
19 Use tobacco products	No	Occasional	<1/2 pack a day	>1 pack a day
20 Drink alcoholic beverages	No	1 per day	2 per day	> 3 per day
21 Number of Doses per Day	1	2	3	4
Total Assessment Score				

Appendix G2:
B-MAAS, Instructions

Over the past several decades, numerous publications have evaluated the factors related to non-adherence. Of course, some of the elements are pretty soft, and others are more robust. When combined, however, these data present a compelling case for identifying which of the thirty-two or so patients you might see today is most likely not to follow their plan of care.

The B-MAAS evaluation criteria have been developed by reviewing Patient Adherence to Treatment: Three Decades of Research. A comprehensive review. By Vermeire, Hearsnhaw, Van Royen, and Denekens, (2001) Journal of Clinical Pharmacy and Therapeutics (2001) 26, 331-342.

Behavioral Education and Research Services, Inc. (BEARS) of Orlando, Florida developed the Green, Yellow, Orange, and Red format of the (BEARS - Medical Adherence Assessment Scale B-MAAS). BEARS' specializes in training programs related to improving patient adherence and staff performance through Adherence Management™. Patients who are evaluated as green or low numbered yellow represent little risk of non-adherence depending upon how the factors are evaluated. Patients in the 19-24 (Yellow) zone are considered to be in the "Mild Risk" category but have crossed the mid-point towards Orange and must be considered and evaluated carefully. Patients in the midrange yellow up through 28 points into the Orange are at medium risk and are considered candidates for more careful consideration. Patients in the Orange level who are greater than 28 and moving into the lower levels of the Red zone are most at risk for non-adherence.

Red zone patients from the midline and above are more likely to have a home health aide or some form of patient care professional who will manage his or her outcome. We have found that patients in the high numbered Red Zone are typically in nursing homes or skilled nursing facilities. Patients in this zone and facing potential discharge before 30 days post-hospital stay need to be carefully transitioned and appropriate supports put in place.

The B-MAAS is best completed by a nurse who has been trained and certified in Adherence Management Coaching early in a hospital or long-term care facility. This information is provided to families so they can understand how patients are identified and selected for inclusion in our Adherence Management program.

Date Assessment Completed:		24-12-14		Total Score:		0	
Name:		John Doe		Risk		Low	
Reviewer:							
Select 1 Level per category based on your assessment and write in the score 0 through 3.	0	1	2	3			
1 Married	Yes	No					
2 Gender	Female	Male	Low Risk	0-12			
			Mild Risk	13-24			
3 Motivated to improve health/condition	Yes	No	Medium Risk	25-36			
			High Risk	>37			
4 Ethnicity	Caucasian	Non-caucasion					

B-MAAS is the screening tool of the Adherence Management Coaching (AdM™ Coaching) Toolkit.

Soft Indicators

The soft indicators are reported in the literature as having some influence on patients and their adherence. These four weak indicators are given only one point each.

Marital Status: The literature supports that people who are married have a higher level of adherence than single people. Non-married individuals should be given a point.

Gender: Historically, women are better at being adherent than males. Because of this difference, males are given a point.

Motivation: This indicator is essential to the overall outcome of the patient and is often the cause for Motivational Interviewing intervention. On initial evaluation, if the impression is one of ambivalence, then a point is given. Patients who express an interest in their outcome will receive no points.

Ethnicity: There is a significant difference between ethnic groups of color. This is particularly true with persons with African American or Hispanic populations. This is due partly to mistrust and partly to a lack of resources or support. This is also prevalent in other countries where one cultural group overshadows other groups.

		College	High School	Middle School	Elementary
5	Education				
0	Age	>80	60-79	40-59	20-49

Education: People with high levels of education tend to be more responsive to the plan of care than people with education levels of high school or lower levels.

Age: Age is inversely related to adherence. For the most part older patients, particularly those who are in their eighth decade are being supported by family members, long-term skilled nursing facilities, or home health services.

		No	Mild	Medium	Severe
7	Vision Impaired				
8	Hearing Impaired	No	Mild	Medium	Severe
9	Memory Impaired	No	Mild	Medium	Severe

Vision impaired: Our concern with visual acuity is related to ensuring that patients can read the materials presented to them or that we may need to make reasonable accommodations to improve their ability.

Hearing-impaired: Hearing acuity has a direct impact on the ability to comprehend instructions related to their care.

Memory impaired: The ability to retain information presented through Teach-Back or other patient education programs has a direct impact on the ability to remember instructions related to their care.

10	Intentional defiance	No	Mild	Medium	Severe
11	Patient/Provider Relationship	>7 visits	5-7	2-4	0-1
12	Medication Side Effects Present	No	Mild	Medium	Severe

Intentional Defiance: Ambivalence or direct defiance because of culture, experience, or personally held beliefs must be considered as a risk indicator if a patient's feelings will interfere with following the plan of care. Intentional defiance needs to be evaluated as a part of the Adherence Improvement Plan (AIP).

Patient/Provider Relationship: The research has consistently indicated that the closer the provider-patient relationship, the higher the likelihood that adherence will follow. Patients who have occasional relationships with one or more providers are less likely to be adherent to the plan of care.

Medication Side Effects Present: Medication side effects such as nausea or drowsiness, represent punishing consequences to patients and increase the likelihood that the patient will abandon the course of therapy. These findings also need to be more closely examined in the AIP.

13	Family Income	High	Medium	Low	None
14	Physical Disability	No	Mild	Medium	Severe
15	Disease Symptoms Present	Severe	Moderate	Mild	No

Family Income: Patients with limited household incomes often have to make economic decisions that are based on disposable income. Expensive medications or even several medications that are prescribed at low co-pays can add up to an unaffordable combination of costs.

Physical Disability: The ability of patients to move around within their homes, manipulate pill bottles or open blister packs will have a negative impact on medication adherence. Additionally, having appropriate transportation to and from the pharmacy will affect acquiring medications.

Disease Symptoms Present: The presence of symptoms can serve as a reminder that patients are in control of their disease and can manage the symptoms through following the plan of care. Typically, patients who have no symptoms are at higher risk of non-adherence than patients with symptoms.

18	Mental Illness Diagnosis/Dementia	No	Mild	Medium	Severe
17	Attitude About Recovery	Good	Moderate	Fair	Bad
18	Understands Disease	Yes	Some	Very little	No

Mental Illness: Mental illness represents a complex set of behavioral problems that need to be specifically addressed. Twenty percent of people have some form of mental illness that can range on the Clinical Global Impression Scale from 2 to 7. One (1) is healthy or not at all ill (Green). Two (2) and three are borderline to mildly ill (Yellow). Four (4) are moderately ill (Orange). Five (5), 6, and 7 range from markedly ill, severely ill, and among the most extremely ill patients (Red).

Attitude about recovery: Patients have a variety of beliefs about an illness that is often culturally or religiously based. Assumptions about their chances for improvement can be influenced by family members, the internet, and many sources. Patients who have a positive attitude about their outcome have a higher likelihood of adherence over those who see the effort as futile or the will of God.

19	Smoke and drink alcohol?	No	Monthly	Weekly	Daily
20	Number of Doses per Day	QD	BID	TID	QID

Understands disease: The more patients understand or want to understand about their condition empowers their ability to want to do something about it. Patients who have a "care-less" attitude about their illness and the methods for management will be at higher risk for non-adherence.

Smoke and drink alcohol: Paired behaviors that have been developed over many years are challenging, but not impossible, to change. People who consume alcohol and smoke daily are at a higher risk of nonadherence than those who combine these behaviors to a lesser degree.

Number of Doses per day: Medication regimen complexity has an impact on adherence. Patients with many prescriptions and have to take them at different times per day are increasingly at risk of either confusion or aggravation. Complex medication regimens tend to take more time and require continuous thinking about which medications need to be taken at what time. How many pills need to be taken? Can they be taken with grapefruit juice, etc.? The greater the degree of aggravation, the higher the probability of non-adherence. Where possible, simplification of the medication regiment must be considered.

Date Assessment Completed	24-12-14		Total Score:	37
Name:	John Doe		Risk	High
Reviewer:	Wright, PhD, RN			
Select 1 Level per category based on your assessment and write in the score 0 through 3.	0	1	2	3

Total Score: When the B-MAAS is completed, the risk factor and final score will be tallied and presented at the top of the page. We believe the B-MAAS needs to be shared with the primary care provider, pharmacy, patient, family, and home health agency to ensure that all people who work with this patient understand that he or she is at high risk for non-adherence.

Appendix H:
BEARS' Physical Ability Assessment Scale (B-PAAS)

Date Assessment Completed:	09 20 2019		Total Score:	0
Name:			Average Score:	0.00
Reviewer:				

Select 1 Level per category based on your assessment and write in the score 1 through 4	0	1	2	3
Physical Ability				
General physical capacity, normally includes the cardio pulmonary, GI, GU, Nervous system, allergic, endocrine, metabolic, nutritional diseases, blood diseases and seizure disorders. Cerebral palsy, GERD, recurrent infections.	Free of any identified or oganic defect or systemic disease.	Presence of stable, minimally signigicant organic defects or systemic diseases (e.g., chronic allergies, well controled diabetes, etc.)	Significant defect(s) or disease(s) under moderate control.	Significant defect(s) or disease(s) have a significant impact on potential and quality of life.
Upper Extremities	L 0 R 0	L R	L R	L R
Concerns spine (cervical and thoracic,) hands, arms in regards to strength, range of motion and general efficiency in use.	Free of any identified or oganic defect or systemic disease.	Slightly limited mobility of joints, mild muscular weakness or other musculoskeletal defects that do not prevent ADLs.	Defect(s) causing moderate interference with functions. Can do some ADLs with support.	Strength, ROM and general efficiency of hands and arms are severely compromsed.
Lower Extremities	L 0 R 0	L R	L R	L R
Concerns the feet, legs pelvic girdle, lower back in regards to strength, range of motion and general efficiency in use	Bones. Muscles, and joints normal.	Slightly limited mobility of joints, mild muscular weakness or other musculoskeletal defects that do not prevent ADLs.	Defect(s) causing moderate interference with functions. Can do some ADLs with support.	Strength, ROM and general efficiency of feet, legs, and pelvic girdle are severely compromsed.
Hearing	L 0 R 0	L R	L R	L R
Concerns the ability for hearing and diseases of the outer and middle ear	Understands whispered instructions (25dB)	Understands normal conversation (65dB).	Moderate hearing loss within the speech frequencies. Understands raised voice.	Profound hearing loss. No measurable hearing in the speech frequencies. No auditory comprehension.
Eyes and Vision	L R	L R	L R	L R
Concerns visual acuity and diseases or defects of the eyes and visual acuity	Reads prescription without glasses.	Reads prescriptions with mild corrective lenses	Reads prescriptions with moderate corrective lenses. Unable to read without glasses.	No measurable vision.
Behavioral	0			
Concerns personality, emotional stability, psychiatric and developmental/intellectual disorders. Psychotropic medications, rumination, self injury, sleep disorders, PICA, battery to others	No impact or potential impact on activities of daily living and safety to self and others, and property.	Little impact or or low risk of impact on activities of daily living and safety to self and others, and property.	Moderate impact or potential impact on activities of daily living and safety to self and others, and property.	Severe impact or potential impact on activities of daily living and safety to self and others, and property.
Communication E	0			
Expressive concerns the ability of patients to share ideas and concerns verbally or through other modalities	Expressive communication has no impact on activities of daily living functions or safety to self and others.	Expressive communication has mild impact on activities of daily living functions or safety to self and others.	Expressive communication has moderate impact on activities of daily living functions or safety to self and others.	Expressive communication has severe impact on activities of daily living functions or safety to
Communication R	0			
Receptive concerns the ability of patients to understand the spoken or written word.	Receptive communication has no impact on activities of daily living functions or safety to self and others.	Receptive communication has mild impact on activities of daily living functions or safety to self and others.	Receptive communication has moderate impact on activities of daily living functions or safety to self and others.	Receptive communication has severe impact on activities of daily living functions or safety to self and others.
Total Assessment Score	0	0	0	0

Appendix I:
ABC Narrative And Training Worksheet

ABC Narrative and Worksheet

1. Whose behavior are you diagramming?_____
2. What is the behavior listed below?_____

(Antecedents) (When this occurs...)	(Behavior) The cues got me thinking...)	(Consequences) If I do or don't do the behavior (These things can occur...)

What Cues led to the behavior you are seeking to increase or decrease?

1. Antecedent Test: List each of the cues that are known to lead to the behavior

2. Environment Test: Is the target behavior okay in some environments but not in others?

3. Related Antecedents Test: Are the cues for behavior related so that one cue may not always lead to the behavior, but two or more cues may come together and result in the target behavior?

What is the targeted behavior you are seeking to increase or decrease?

1. Pet Rock Test: Get a rock and make it your pet. If your pet rock can do the behavior perfectly then it is not a behavior (e.g., sit quietly).

2. Does the behavior involve doing something (e.g., talking, touching walking, swallowing). Behavior is what a person says or does.

What are the consequences that follow the behavior you are seeking to increase or decrease?

1. Positive or Negative for the behavior? (P/N)

2. During or After the Behavior? (I/F) Reinforcement or punishment while doing the behavior (Immediate) is more powerful than a consequence that occurs in the future.

3. Likely/Unlikely (L/U) Consequences that have a high degree of likelihood are more reliable than consequences that are unlikely to occur.

4. Aware/Not aware (A/N) Consequences that are not perceived by the patient do not have the same effect as consequences they are aware of.

Behavior Analysis Worksheet

A. Whose behavior are you diagramming? _____

B. What is the behavior you are diagramming? _____

C. What is the setting where the behavior occurs? _____

D. Is the behavior acceptable any where else? _____

ANTECEDENT (Cue)	BEHAVIOR (TARGET)	CONSEQUENCES
What happened before the Bx?	What was the behavior?	What happened after the Bx?

©BEARS 2014

Index

A

Adherence Improvement Plan viii, 3, 10
  Accountability 135
  Lifestyle Change 136
  Measuring 110
  Outcomes 109
  Page Two 113
  Pinpoints 109
  Reinforcement Plan 115
  Target Behavior 113
  Team Effort 112
Adherence Management Coaching 7, 9
AdM Coach
  Advanced 4
  Basic 3
  Evidence Based 9
  Intermediate 3
  Team
    Nurses, pharmacist, transition care 10
  When Things Are Not Working 132
AdM Home Coach ix, xi, 1, 3, 4, 10, 119, 120, 121, 128, 136
  Certified 2
  Emotions 121
  Investment 138
  Patient Interaction 121
Affordable Care Act 2010 vii
Aggression 17
Antecedent 5, 113, 116, 117, 119, 135, 140
Applied Behavior Analysis 1, 9
Aristotle 5, 134
Audiologist i
Autism 1

B

BEARS Adherence Consequence Analysis (BACA) viii, 145, 146
BEARS Medical Adherence Assessment Survey B-MAAS 9, 158
BEARS Physical Abilities Assessment Survey B-PAAS 10
Behavior 14
  Adherent ix, xi, 19
  Baseline 116
  Compliant 19
  Consequences 11
  Desired Behavior 19
  Examples 14
  Flawlessly Execute 12
  Labels 17
  Lindsley's Definition 14
  Non-adherence 9
  Non-adherent vii, 9
  Shape, Correct, Reinforce 138
  Starting and Maintaining 116
  Stop-Redirect-Reinforce 127

C

CABG iv
Care Plan vii, 10, 12
Categories of Learning
  Conscious Competence-Mastery xi
  Conscious Incompetence-Awareness x
  Unconscious Competence-Fluency xi
  Unconscious Incompetence-Ignorant Bliss x
CCU iv
Cherry Picking ii
Cheshire Cat viii
Clinical Tasks 12

Cognitive Behaviorists 14
Common Sense 5
Conflicting signals vii
Consequence
  Abandoned viii
  Care Plan viii
  Clinical viii
  Extinction 138
  Negative 118
  Perception (Aware or Not Aware)
    118
  PFLN 114
  PILA 114
  Punishers vii, x
  Punishing viii
Consistency 2
Cultural Stewpot 6

D

Daniels, Aubrey i, 9
  Behavior-Based Safety 130
  Performance Management 9, 130,
    141
Dead Person Test 16
Dickinson, Emily 14
Discharge Checklist viii
Dr. Stein. *See* Stein, Michael

E

Employee Assistance Programs (EAP)
  131
Extubated vi

F

Family Involvement ix
Fluent ix

H

Habit i, iii, viii, xi, 1, 4, 5, 6, 7, 8, 9, 10,
    12, 13, 16, 18, 112, 116, 117,
    119, 121, 130, 132, 133, 135,
    136, 138, 140
Healthcare Culture 6
Heart cath iv

Hippocrates vii, 130
Home Caregiver 2
Home Healthcare Team ix

L

Lemon Dropping ii
Lovaas, Ivar 131, 134

M

Medication Therapy Management 7
Mixed signals vii
Motivational Interviewing 7, 14

O

O2 concentrators viii
Old Habits ix
Outcomes viii, 2, 7, 16, 18, 109, 115,
    133, 155
  Celebrate 115
  Clinical 134
  Define 115
  Desired 132
  Measure 112
  Planned 118
  Unwanted 138

P

Past Performance 136
Patient ii, iii, vi, vii, viii, ix, xi, 2, 7, 9,
    10, 12, 13, 16, 17, 18, 19, 20,
    106, 107, 108, 109, 110, 112,
    113, 114, 115, 117, 118, 119,
    120, 121, 122, 123, 124, 125,
    126, 127, 128, 129, 130, 131,
    132, 133, 134, 135, 136, 138,
    139, 140, 152, 153, 154, 155,
    159, 161, 162, 165
  Adherence 7
  Education iii, v

R

Recording Data 11
Reinforcement

Bribery 113
Intermittent viii
Reinforcer
   Positive (R+) x, 113
   Ratio 138
Results viii, xi, 1, 12, 16, 18, 111, 129,
       132, 133, 135, 136, 152, 155

S

Samuel Clemmons. *See* Twain, Mark
Skilled Nursing Facility (SNF) viii
Social Constructs 6
Stein, Michael 107, 108, 112, 113, 116,
       151, 152
   Patient Beatriz 107, 111, 112, 113,
       151, 152, 154
      AIP 150
      BACA 149
Stents ii

T

Teachback 7
The Science of Behavior 1, 2, 3, 7, 134,
       135, 136, 138
Transitional Care Nurse viii, 132, 139
Transitional Care Team 17
Troponin ii
Truth or Consequences 137
Twain, Mark iii
   Habit is Habit iii, 16

U

Unhealthy habits 11

W

Why is that important? 11
Wright, Bob 1
Wright, Jefferson v
Wright, Jude Ann v
Wright-Lindsley Matrix 10
Wright-Lindsley Model 128

What's Your NEXT STEP? Telehealth!

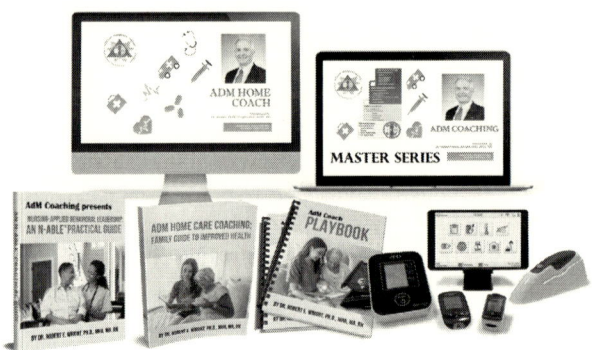

HOME CARE AND TELEHEALTH IS
NOW THE NEW NORMAL.

BEARS and AdM Coaches have partnered with Dictum Health to bring you the nex1 generation of Telehealth care. Our Home Care Bundle includes Dictum Health's Remote Patient Monitoring (RPM) and Chronic Care Management (CCM) Devices, along with the AdM Home Coach Certification Series.

Dictum Health is advancing new methods for home-based care using the integration of videoconferencing with the simultaneous streaming of vital-signs, cardiopulmonary data, and medical images. From the Virtual Exam Room (VER) remote clinicians can conduct a VER with a patient for a complete clinical examination to assess, diagnose, and recommend treatment with the accuracy of an in-hospital exam.

Real-time remote patient assessment using Bluetooth-enabled FDA approved medical devices (such as blood pressure, SpO2, blood sugar, temperature, and weight) enables a care team, or clinician, to respond rapidly to any change in health status. Clinical home monitoring with Dictum Health's end-to-end telehealth system supports care coordination and improves patient engagement, while allowing patients, to continue their treatment and stay connected with their care team from home.

Patients or their caregivers can now be sent home with the Dictum Health home kit to provide greater confidence and support in managing their chronic condition, recovering from surgery, or completing their care plan. Meanwhile, the patient's clinician, or AdM Coach Care Team, can track the patient's progress in Care Central Cloud Services with live updates on the patient's vital signs, cardiopulmonary status, and other health data.

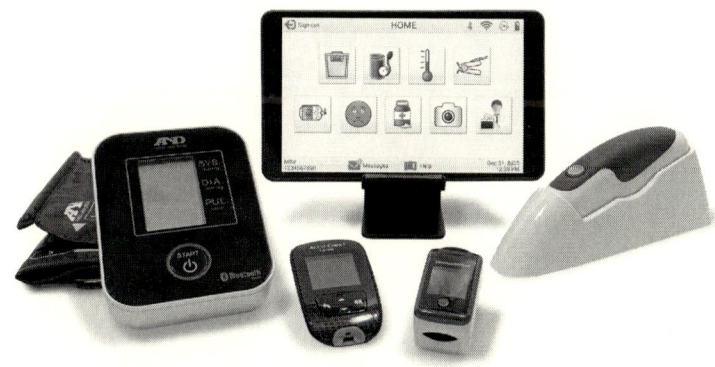